BODY C

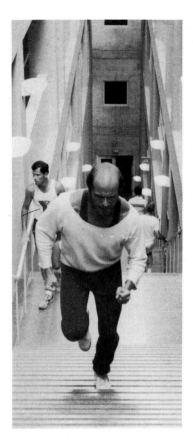

ACKNOWLEDGEMENTS

Special thanks to Al Green for writing the Aerobics section and assisting with the stretch.

Thank you to the Central Toronto YMCA and Gold's Gym in Toronto for use of their facilities for photography purposes.

Thank you to Colours for doing the ladies' colours and make-up and David Alexander for hair design.

DEDICATION
To my Dad.

First published by Summerhill Press Limited, Toronto, Ontario.
First UK edition published by Patrick Stephens Limited, Wellingborough, Northamptonshire, 1988.

Photography: John Porter
Editor: Jim Christie
Design: Design Force, Brian Moore
Illustrations: Francis Key Kupka

British Library Cataloguing in Publication Data

Turner, Roger L.
  Body culture.
  1. Exercise   2. Physical fitness
  I. Title   II. Green Al
  613.7'1   RA781

ISBN 1-85260-085-3

Patrick Stephens is part of the Thorsons Publishing Group, Wellingborough, Northamptonshire, NN8 2RQ, England.

Printed and bound in Great Britain by Butler & Tanner Ltd, Frome and London

10 9 8 7 6 5 4 3 2

BODY CULTURE

BY ROGER L. TURNER

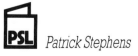 Patrick Stephens

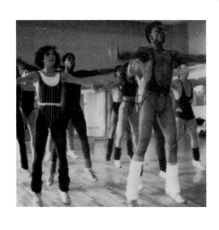

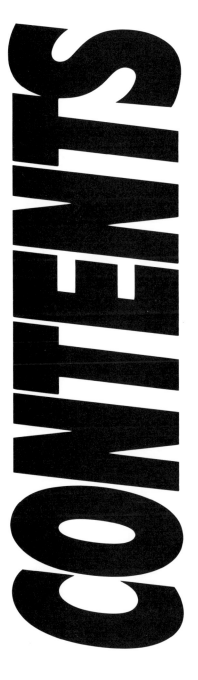

CONTENTS

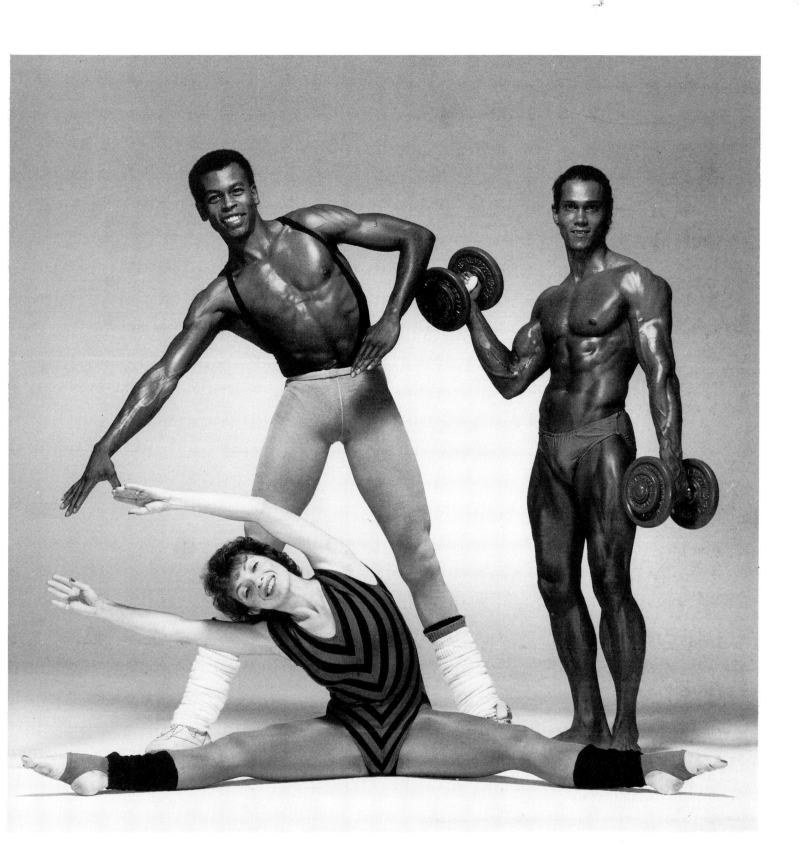

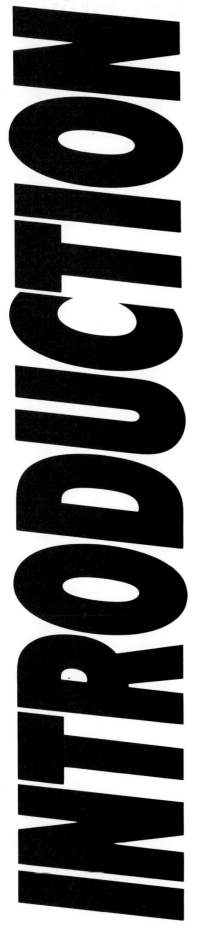

INTRODUCTION

*W*ELCOME TO BODY CULTURE.

*W*elcome to the total approach to fitness.

*T*his is the book that combines science with common sense to blend three fundamental types of exercise into programs for you to reach your physical potentials.

*I*t is a map which will help you identify your fitness goal and show you the path for attaining that goal. The models we have used in this book are not hired, professional posers. They are ordinary people, such as yourself, who set goals for themselves. We have included their biographies and training information to illustrate realistically for the reader what can be accomplished with various programs over a certain period of time.

*I*n *Body Culture*, the exercises have been arranged according to the specific body parts they affect. This facilitates comparison, allows easy reference and aids in establishing rehabilitation programs for specific injuries.

*T*he emphasis in each exercise is always on the form of execution. The book contains detailed explanations of the moves, with accompanying pictures and suggested variations for certain exercises.

*C*are has been taken to explain the major contributory elements of intensity and discipline in training — the psychological necessities of a complete program.

*S*pecial chapters have also been written on fitness for children; exercises for the prevention and rehabilitation of back problems; exercises that can be done when travelling away from home.

*W*e all have fitness goals, whether we consciously admit them or not. A simple glance into a mirror, or a stroll along the beach is usually enough to remind us that no one is perfect. There is always some part of our bodies that we wish was larger, or smaller, or stronger.

Body Culture's extensive section on weight training helps you to isolate the muscle groups that need the extra work to be come proportionate and more defined. Also, the strength gains will enhance athletic performance and help reduce the incidence of injury.

*T*here isn't one of us who hasn't wished at one time or another that he had more energy or endurance. The aerobic component of your exercise program will give your body its necessary cardiovascular training effect. The more efficiently your body uses oxygen, the more energy you have.

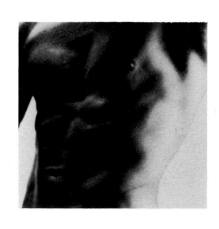

The section on stretches has a dual purpose. First, stretching of muscles before and after workouts helps prevent muscle soreness which might discourage continuation of a training program. Secondly, the same stretches also prevent the muscles from contracting and shortening with age. Stretching will maintain and gradually increase your flexibility.

Body Culture *leads you through the beginner's basics to the advanced level of exercise, allowing you to combine the three components of your fitness program as they are best suited to your own goals.*

The one thing this book does not offer you is a miracle. There are no short cuts to physical fitness, no quick fixes. A body gets out of shape over a length of time and it will take a proportionate amount of time to bring it to superb condition.

But the rewards are worth it. It is satisfying and fulfilling to set goals, strive for them and finally attain your potential, creating a masterpiece of human sculpture.

That's something to celebrate.

*And that's **Body Culture**.*

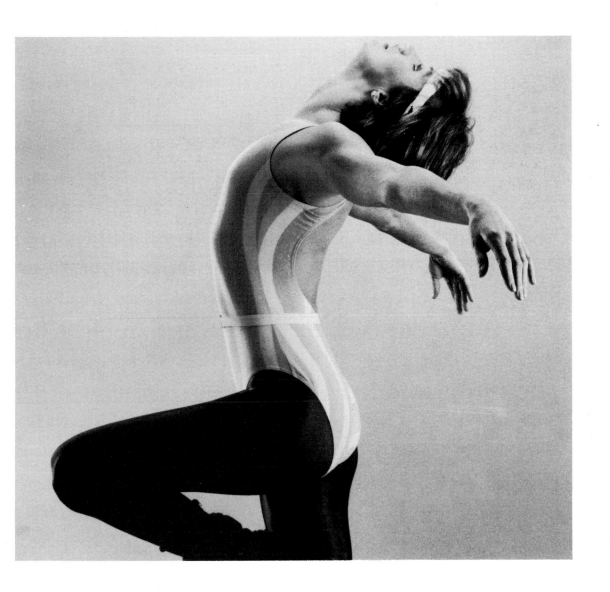

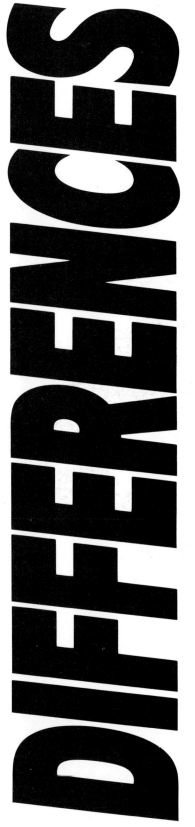

DIFFERENCES

Many people have the mistaken impression that there are fundamental physiological differences between men and women that require them to have absolutely different exercise programs.

Yet, as I studied anatomy at college, it became apparent to me that male and female musculature is the same. The origin, insertion and function of the muscles is identical in both sexes. The main difference consists of muscle size and a higher capacity for strength among men than women.

The form (execution) and the relative effect of each exercise we will present is the same for both sexes in each discipline. The variables will be time, intensity, the number of repetitions and the amount of weight used – but form remains the same.

Consequently, when designing exercise programs for men or for women, the exercises chosen will be determined acording to your goal, not your sex.

Any person wishing to increase strength, muscle size and definition and to cut down body fat would concentrate mostly on weights, inclusive of pre- and post-exercise stretches to prevent muscle shortening. The program also would include some aerobic activity to burn off calories and to train the cardiovascular system.

Women generally have a slightly higher content of body fat than do men, and therefore, the aerobic component of their workout is greater than that for men.

Men and women train well together. Women generally can do more intense workouts for longer periods of time, while men can usually lift heavier weights. Each draws encouragement to improve from the other's abilities. There is a desire to progress to the training partner's level in either duration or weight.

WOMEN'S FEARS

The excuse I hear most frequently from women who do not want to undertake a strenuous exercise or weight training program is that they do not want to wind up with a physique like some professional female body builders and large Olympic athletes.

A woman simply does not get that type of body unless she resorts to using anabolic steroids and male hormones.

When a woman exercises with weights she becomes a little stronger and much more shapely. To create even a modest amount of musculature on a woman is a long, slow process, but she cannot obtain big muscles without the use of steroids.

A drug-free workout program will make your muscles stronger, shaplier and more defined. These changes won't happen overnight. They are small, and progressive and it will take time to reform your body to the shape you want.

MEN'S DISAPPOINTMENT

Many men start out weight training and expect phenomenal gains in a year or less. They get disappointed when, after much hard work, they have smaller measurements. What has happened is that their body fat has decreased, disappearing not only from the obvious areas, but from between muscle fibres.

Your measurements may be smaller at first, but you have gained healthy muscle tissue and lost dangerous fat accumulations. Don't turn to dangerous steroids as a shortcut to faster gains. Put smaller measurements in the right perspective: not smaller, but with less fat content.

Unless you are in your teens or early 20s, nature dictates slow, progressive gains. But, with persistent training, attention to diet, sufficient rest and time, you can change the way you look without drugs. There is a feeling of pride in knowing that the gains came from your own discipline and dedication and not from a bottle or injection.

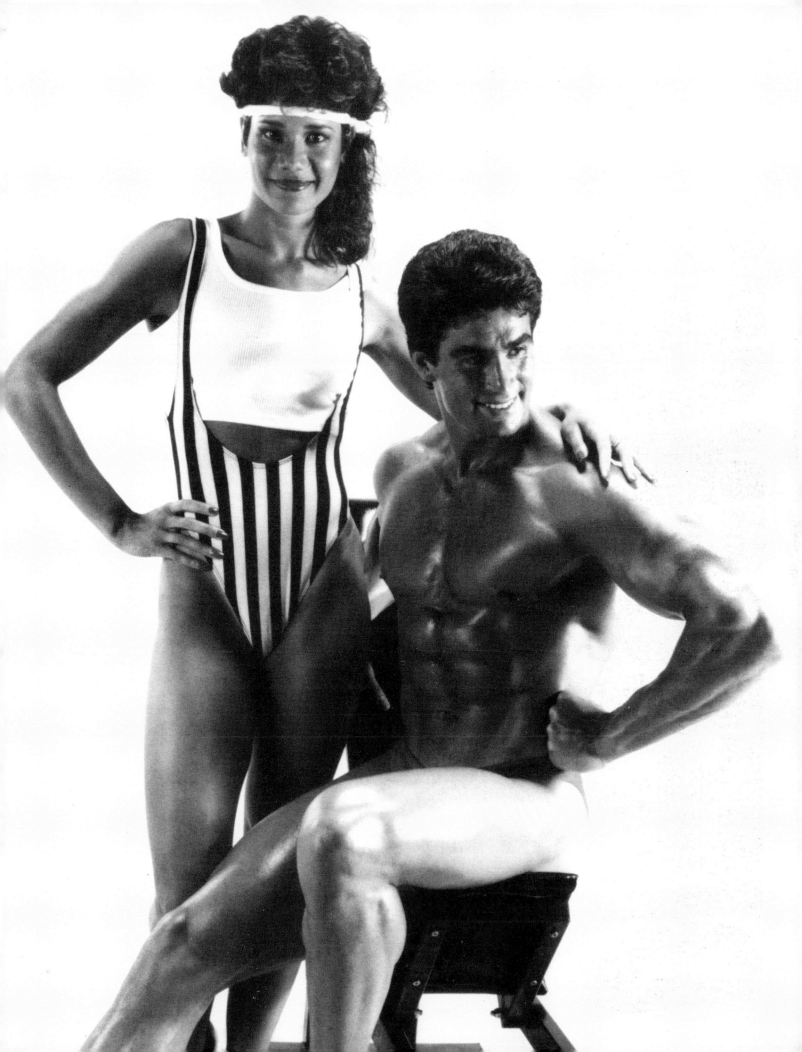

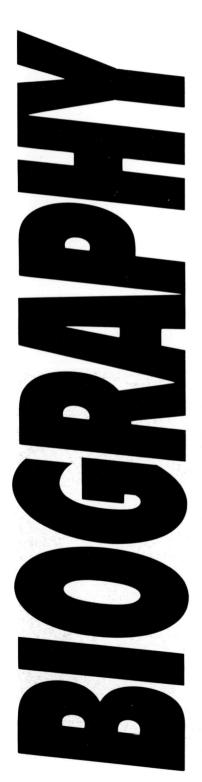

BIOGRAPHY

Roger Turner, 39.
Author; Chiropractor, Father, Director Rosedale Chiropractic Group, Toronto. Enjoys weight training, squash, aerobics, windsurfing

Has trained with weights since February, 1981. Currently on a three-day split program. Tuesday – legs, shoulders, abdominals, calves; Thursday – chest, back, abdominals; Saturday – biceps, triceps, abdominals. Workouts include stationary bike warm-up and specific stretches for muscles used. Sunday – aerobics class.

"Pick the exercise that helps you accomplish your goal. Combine it with the other disciplines and be consistent and persistent with your workouts. Have a long term goal for your health with many short-term fitness goals along the way."

Alvin Greene, 30.
Owner-operator of Body Alive Studios Ltd. Enjoys basketball, baseball, horseback riding, cycling, football, soccer, karate, judo. Has been dancing jazz and ballet in Toronto, New York, Boston, Chicago and Washington since 1974.

Main forms of exercise are aerobics and dance, six days per week, two classes a day – one hour of workout and one hour of stretching. Also cycles six miles per day, to and from work.

"The reason for exercise is not only for a long life, but a better quality of life, a sharper mind and improved skills in all physical activities."

Tracey Tanner, 25.
Fitness instructor and dancer. Enjoys aerobics, dance and weight training. Has been working out for 10 years and exercises six to seven times per week.

Goal is to maintain a low percentage of body fat and to have a body that is well defined and well toned. Wants to reach ultimate levels in the three fitness components – strength, flexibility and endurance.

"Fitness and exercise is as important to the body as is rest and proper nutrition. We make the time to eat and sleep and we must also do it for exercise. Life is not complete without it. It's essential for a totally healthy lifestyle."

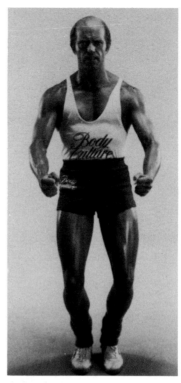

Roger Turner

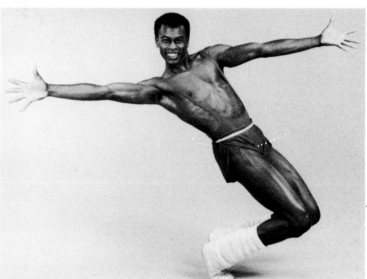

Alvin Green

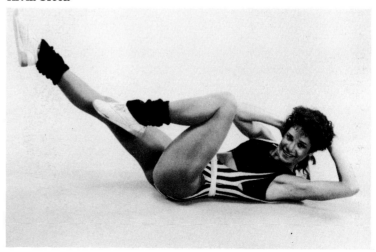

Tracey Tanner

Lloyd Adams, 23.
Dancer. Enjoys ballet, jazz, gymnastics and aerobics. Dance and aerobics provide the bulk of training program.

Has been involved in aerobics and gymnastics for approximately 14 years; dance for four and a half years.

"My goal with exercise has been to stay strong and healthy. Exercise enables one to live a longer and healthier life."

Rhys Berthiaume, 28.
Model, actor, fitness instructor. Enjoys aerobics, cycling, swimming, jazz dancing, volleyball, basketball, weightlifting and stretching.

Teaches five to six aerobics and stretching classes per week, participates in three others. Involved in aerobics for 18 months. Also cycles and swims for exercise three to four times per week. Goals are to maintain a high level of fitness while building strength and endurance; to develop an inner physical awareness and to improve athletic abilities.

"Fitness is having the strength and endurance to go about daily activities without exhaustion. Exercise is important in strengthening muscular and cardiovascular endurance, decreasing chance of muscle injury, providing an emotional release and increased self-confidence."

Wendy Sanham, 24.
Dancer and teacher. Enjoys ballet and jazz dancing, aerobics, swimming, skiing, windsurfing and team sports.

Has been involved in fitness pursuits for 14 years and has aerobic workouts six to seven times per week.

"My goal is simply to be as healthy as I can be. 'Mens sana in corpore sano' – a healthy mind in a healthy body."

Pam Fraser, 23.
Bank teller, Hamilton, Ont. Enjoys weight training and body building. Has been lifting weights seriously for two years.

Program includes 200 repetitions of abdominal exercises every morning and two-hour workouts six days a week, concentrating on different body parts each workout.

"It takes time. You have to be patient and put the hours in to get the results you want."

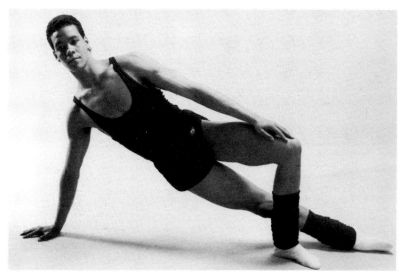

Lloyd Adams

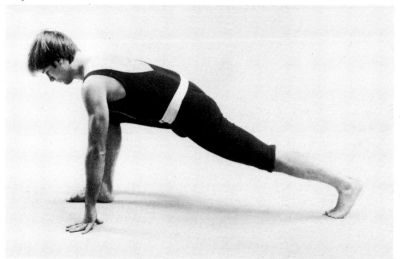

Rhys Berthiaume

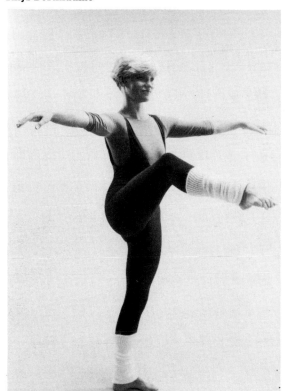

Wendy Sanham

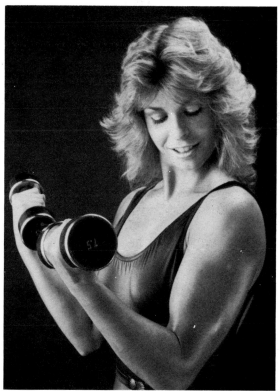

Pam Fraser

Lee Bristow, 29

Advertising agency creative assistant, and also aerobics class instructor. Her exercise program consists of teaching aerobics and stretching classes three times per week, taking two dance classes per week, and weight training twice weekly.

Her goals are to maintain a low level of body fat, and at the same time a high level of fitness.

"I feel that success in business can be enhanced with exercise and diet combined with a positive mental attitude."

Paul Robbins, 29.

Owner-manager of a steel company. Enjoys cycling, running, swimming, windsurfing and skiing. Competes in triathlon.

Combines morning weight training with aerobic exercise after work. Program – two-day split: first day, chest, shoulders, back, abdominals; second day, biceps, legs, triceps, abdominals. Works out four times per week in summer, six times per week in winter. Cycles and swims twice a week, runs three times a week.

"Fitness has to be your lifestyle. It's not just a matter of making one hour for your workout. Eating habits and rest must revolve around it as well. The goal is long-term – where is it going to get you in 20 years?

Louise Calvert, 37.

Housewife, fitness coordinator and instructor. Enjoys squash and skiing. Has been working out seriously for the past three years. Teaches 10 classes per week and plays squash or skis twice a week.

"The keys to fitness is to maintain a positive attitude and to stick with it. It is something you must do for yourself and it must be a lifetime thing. It's tough to get people to commit themselves. People want to spend three months to get in shape and hope it will last them five years."

Rico Dividio, 23

Fitness instructor and consultant, and weight training model. Has been a body builder for five years. He works out six days a week for 2-3 hours per day.

His routine consists mainly of weight training with a split of two different body parts each day plus the abs, and over 30 minutes on a stationary bicycle for aerobics.

"My goal is to continue my muscle growth to gain more muscle definition. I take it one day at a time, and I know the harder I work out the more it pays off."

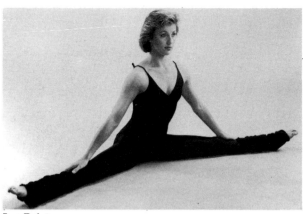

Lee Bristow

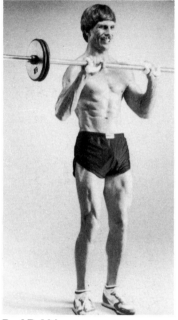

Paul Robbins

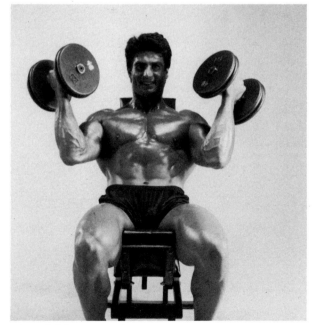

Louise Calvert

Rico Dividio

Rebecca Bell, 21.
Fitness instructor and consultant, fitness writer, Bachelor of Fine Arts – dance. Enjoys aerobics, cross-country skiing, cycling, swimming, running, kayaking, sailing and skating.

Has been seriously concerned with fitness for 10 years and has taught aerobics for five. Workouts six days per week, teaching seven classes and participating in three to four more (basically stretching). Also runs three miles, twice a week. Fitness goals include low percentage of body fat, high cardiovascular endurance, toned muscles and good flexibility.

"High standards for health and exercise make for high standards in all other areas of life. Exercise should be enjoyable, rewarding and include challenge."

Sherry Heise, 23.
Marketing coordinator, Hamilton, Ont. Former gymnast, training in body building for the past year. Combines weight training, aerobics and stretch in a comprehensive program.

Weight training – chest, back, biceps, two times a week; legs, shoulders, triceps, two times a week; calves and abdominals, each three times a week. Aerobics – stationary bike, 25 km in one hour, four times a week. Stretch – full body, 15 to 30 minutes daily.

"Since age 13, I've had to watch my diet. The key has been to watch what I eat, combined with a consistent exercise program. I prefer weights for the quickest, most visible results."

Patrick Truyens, 26.
Engineering technician. Has enjoyed bodybuilding and a multiplicity of sports for many years. Has been a bodybuilder for two years, working 75 per cent of the time on free weights, the remainder on Nautilus equipment. Exercises three to four times per week, up to two hours per session.

"Total fitness is not a fad or a flash in the pan. I made a commitment to myself years ago not to allow myself to fall apart. It takes hard work and patience, but it's gratifying to see the results."

Brenda Reinbolt, 24.
Professional dancer. Enjoys tennis, volleyball, baseball. Exercise types include aerobics, ballet, jazz and modern dance.

Works out daily and has been involved seriously in aerobic exercise for the past two and a half years. Goal has been to look strong and healthy, so that strength is reflected in her dancing and her career will last longer.

"Through health and exercise, one will feel better about himself or herself and live a longer and happier life."

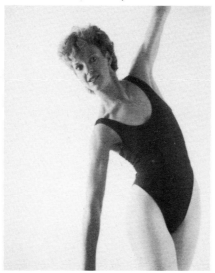

Rebecca Bell

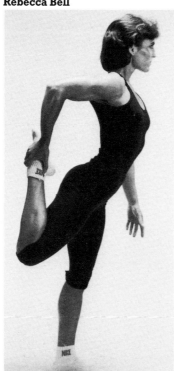
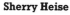

Sherry Heise

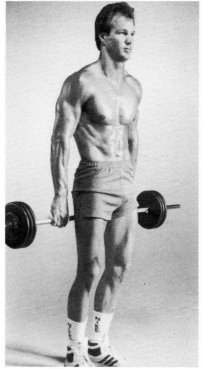

Patrick Truyens

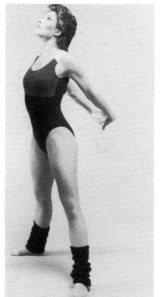

Brenda Reinbolt

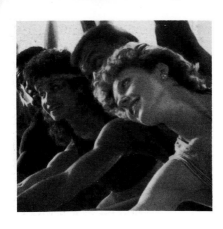

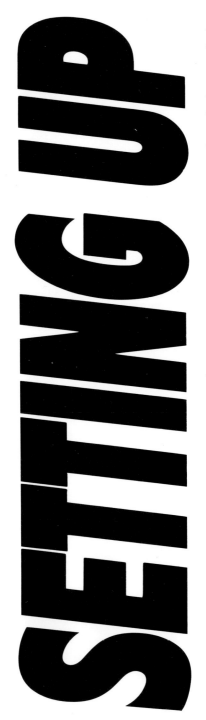

Once you have established a fitness goal, you need to know how to combine different exercises to achieve that end. All of us need strength, flexibility and aerobic exercise to achieve and maintain our fitness and health goals. The goal itself determines where you place the emphasis in your exercise program. Whatever your goal, it can be achieved by following the principles outlined in **Body Culture.**

COMMON GOALS

LOSING WEIGHT:

This is the most common goal for people beginning an exercise program and we have included a chapter dealing specifically with weight loss. The objective of losing weight is to decrease body fat, while at the same time increasing your endurance, flexibility and strength. The emphasis is on diet, as explained in the chapter on weight loss, and on aerobic exercise, which is the most efficient way to burn calories.
Weight training and stretching are not directly connected to weight loss and, therefore, are de-emphasized at this stage. Weight loss is simple arithmetic – you need to burn up more calories than you consume.

INCREASED ENERGY:

This second most common fitness goal is especially popular among business people. The stress of their daily routines and lack of exercise, combined with irregular meals and junk food or fast food leads to chronic fatigue.

A common mistake is to eat more to get more energy. For anyone not involved in physical activity, this results in more fat storage and an actual decrease energy because there is more weight to cart around.

Any of the three forms of exercise will contribute to an increase in energy. Simply getting the body active regularly raises the metabolism. You will find that the more you do, the more you can do.

So often, we hear the complaint "I just don't have the energy to exercise." But those who make the effort discover the increase in energy is almost immediate. When the exercise is discontinued, the energy level drops off right away. This is the reason why most of us involved in fitness are "hooked" on regular exercise. If we stop, we feel much less energetic.

Any exercise at this stage is beneficial. Start with whatever is easiest – if it's enjoyable, you're more likely to continue on a regular basis – then work on toward your goals.

INCREASED ENDURANCE:

Your endurance refers to your ability to maintain activity for an extended period of time; to last; to continue.

To achieve this goal, aerobics is the key. Start off in a beginner's aerobics class and progress to more strenuous levels as your endurance improves. Other aerobic activities to consider include running (or games that involve running), cycling, swimming and cross-country skiing.

To achieve an aerobic training effect, these activities must be done continuously for a minimum of 20 minutes at 70% to 80% of your maximum heart rate, at least three times per week. Your target zone is calculated by subtracting your age from 220, then multiplying the result by .70 or .80.

An example, using my age:
$(220 - 39) \times .80 = 144.8$

So, my heart needs to beat about 145 times per minute, for 20 minutes, three times per week for me to obtain benefit from aerobic exercise.

Fat is used as the energy source during this process, whereas the body's glycogen stores are used for energy in weight training.

FIRMING UP:

To start firming up requires a combination of aerobics and weight training. Many of our models in the book have firmed up very nicely by using only aerobics or only weights. However, the best results are achieved by using the aerobics to burn off fat and to increase endurance, while using the weights to fully utilize the muscles and to change the body's shape. This leads to a firmer, more attractive appearance.

Body Culture focuses on specific body parts to help you with target areas.

SPOT REDUCING:

Spot reducing is a misnomer, because losing excess fat by ityself, in one particular area is not possible. Consider trying to take a scoop of water out of one corner of a bucket. The water level is reduced over all, but the place from which the water was taken still looks like every other place in the bucket. The same applies to body fat. To reduce fat areas that are a particular problem, the over all fat content of the body must be reduced.

However, these fatty deposits can serve a purpose. We all have a specific area of the body where fat seems to accumulate. Mine sits on the sides of my waist. For you, it may be the hips or buttocks. Use these fatty areas as a monitor to indicate when to decrease your calorie intake and when to increase your aerobic exercise.

Exercises for a specific body part will help to tone the muscle in that area, but will not necessarily reduce fat there.

INCREASING MUSCLE SIZE:

Muscle size increases come from progressive resistance weight training. It must be emphasized that quality of muscle size is important. You can get bigger all over by taking in more calories than are necessary, but this is a fat increase, not a quality muscle increase.

When I first started weight training, the size of my chest increased four inches in the first two months. A tailor had to let out my vests. But as my training progressed, the quality of my muscle fibre increased, with less fat and water interspersed with the muscle tissue. My measurements went down, almost to where they were at the beginning. That could have been very disappointing if I hadn't posed for pictures at six-month intervals. They showed the truth – that the progress was considerable and dramatic.

INCREASING STRENGTH:

This will come from weight training, done on a progressive basis, using lower repetitions, fewer sets and increasingly heavier weights. Record-keeping, on a per workout basis, is essential to tell you when you are ready to increase your weights.
Example: Bench press – After a light warm-up set, start with a weight that you can lift for only six repetitions and no more. Do three sets. If the weight is 180 pounds, note this in your records as 180 – 3 x 6. On the next workout, strive for one more repetition with the same weight, 180 – 3 x 7. Once you can do nine to 10 repetitions, then add five per cent more weight, or as much weight as you can lift for six repetitions.

FLEXIBILITY:

Unfortunately, flexibility is not as popular a goal as some of the others because most of us don't realize how important it is.
One must realize that, as we get older, our muscles naturally shrink and get shorte. This decreases our range of motion and eventually even hinders regular daily activities.

Incorporating stretching into my regular exercise program made a tremendous difference in my ability to perform the exercises I ususally do, as well as decreasing the muscle soreness after workouts. To some athletes, flexibility is essential to the performance of their sports. To the rest of us, it is essential to slow down the aging process. Stretching exercises should be included in everyone's exercise program.

SPECIFICS:

The above goals can be broken down into specific looks or body types or specializations for local muscle groups.
A person, for example, may have genetically small calves, compared with the rest of his bodily proportions. If he is concerned with getting them up to par with the rest of his body, he would concentrate on weight training exercises specific to the calf muscle.

Examples of different exercise programs and their results are found in the biographies of the models used in this book.
The cross-section of different body types and combinations is interesting, as are the details on frequency of workouts and the number of years in training. You can obtain some idea what it will take to achieve the look you like.

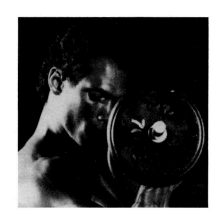

WEIGHTS

DEFINITION:

Weight training is a form of exercise performed using a weighted object (barbell, dumbell or exercise machine) to provide resistance to the normal range of motion of a particular body part. The resistance is provided to increase the amount of effort required by a particular muscle or muscle group, to move a joint through its full range of motion. When done in a progressive program, the muscle adapts over time, by growing stronger to handle the increased demands placed upon it.

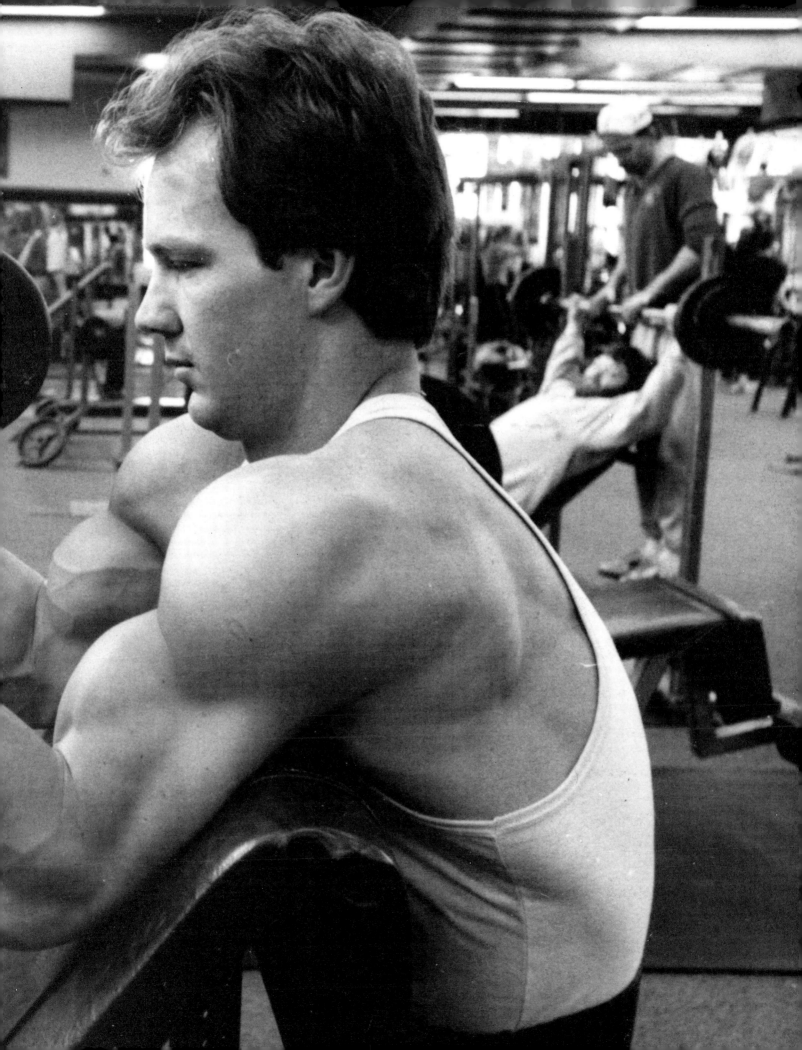

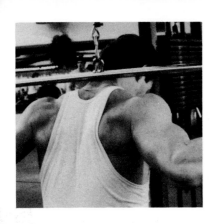

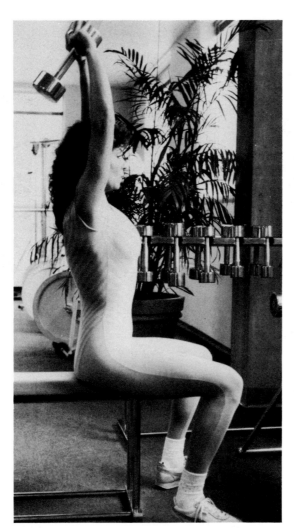

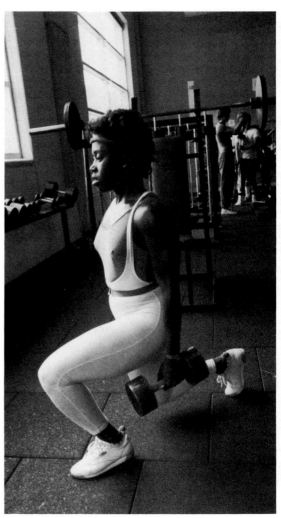

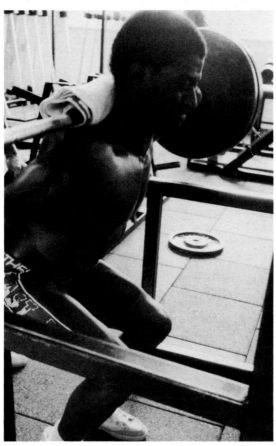

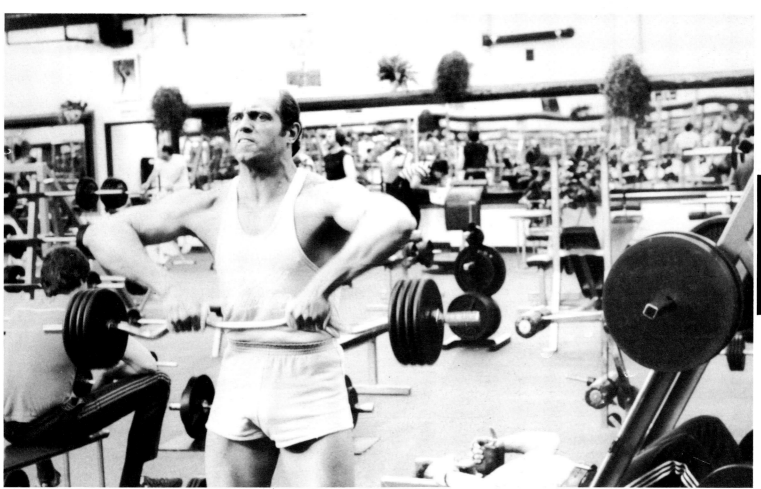

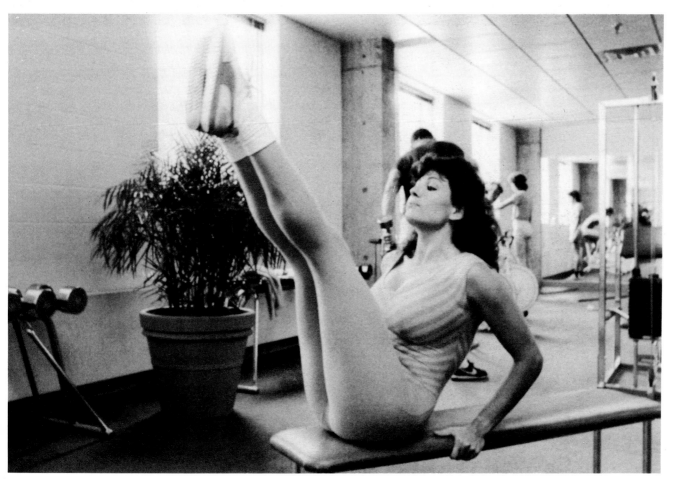

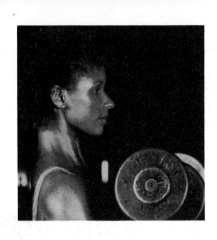

*F*orm is the most important word in the vocabulary of weight training. Form for each exercise entails a very precise order of movements with a weight, through a specific range of motion, always maintaining complete control. Each exercise has been recommended because of its focus upon a particular muscle or muscle group.

*C*orrect form stresses these muscles safely and maximizes gains. Consider correct form for the bicep exercise of dumbell curls. As an experiment, place your left hand on the right bicep; hold the right arm down at your side with the fist clenched, fingers against the thigh. With your hand in this position, flex the arm at the elbow to full flexion. Notice the extent of the contraction of the bicep. Now, supinate the hand (ie. turn the fist palm-up) and notice that the contraction of the bicep has increased. It is a graphic example of how proper form maximizes the benefit of each exercise.

*T*o ignore form is to deny yourself maximum benefit and to risk injury. Correct form can help prevent ligament and tendon tears, muscle spasms, sprains, fractures, subluxations, backaches, cracked ribs and knee problems.

*D*o not sacrifice form for heavier weights, a longer workout or more apparent stretch. It won't improve your results and it may take weeks to recover the injuries that result from poor form.

*S*ome examples of common pitfalls to avoid in weight training: swinging the weight, so that it moves by momentum, rather than by controlled contraction; using other muscle groups to perform an exercise; performing an exercise at the incorrect angle; using too heavy a weight that prevents full range of motion; arching the back; jerking the knees; performing the exercise too fast, allowing the weight to drop, rather than lowering it under control; swaying back and forth.

A note on speed of performance. Your speed can determine the amount of stress on a particular muscle or group. Slow repetitions keep resistance on the muscle through its range of motion for a longer time. The preferred pace is to take two to three seconds to raise the weight, then three to four seconds to lower it. Keep it slow and controlled.

*I*t is also advisable to vary your pace regularly (a little faster or slower) to avoid allowing the muscles to become accustomed to the routine.

*D*on't be afraid to sacrifice weight for form. You can always increase the intensity of the workout by increasing the number of repetitions. But too heavy a weight, improperly lifted, will neither isolate nor fully develop the muscles you want to work on.

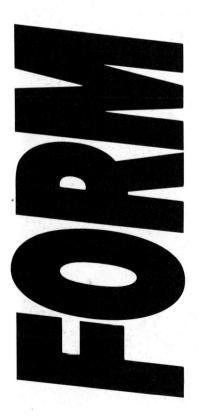

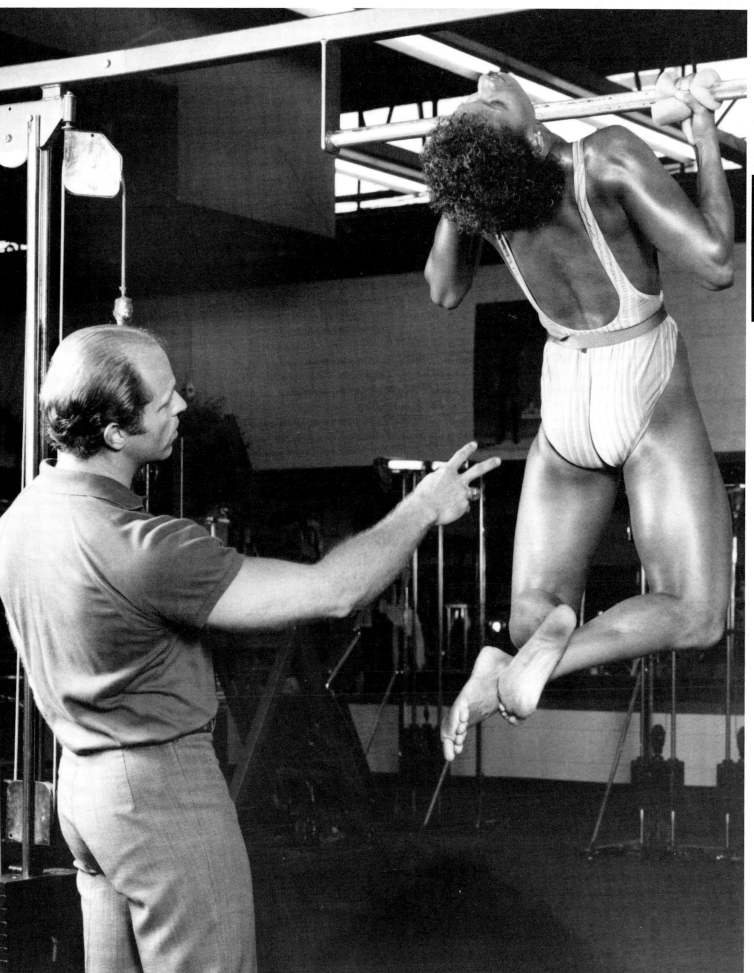

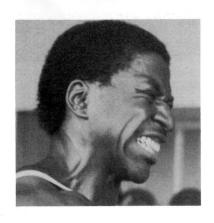

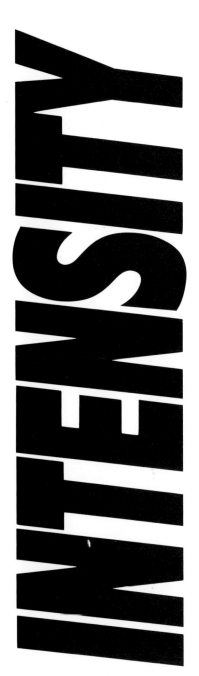

Intensity is composed of concentration on the form of the exercise, the amount of effort utilized to perform the exercise and the duration of the effort.

For example, three people are asked to move equal piles of wood from Point A to Point B. The first person takes one hour to move his pile of wood, piece by piece. The second moves the pile in 15 minutes. The third person uses a machine and moves the entire pile at once, in one minute.

The second person's effort is obviously the most physically intense of the three. Even though the third person accomplishes the task faster, his personal effort is minimal. Likewise, to increase the intensity of your workouts, it is necessary to increase the amount of effort expended.

This can be done along three dimensions:
1. Increase the amount of weight to be lifted in each exercise (though not past the point where form suffers).
2. Increase the number of repetitions for a particular exercise.
3. Decrease the amount of time it takes to perform the same number of sets and repetitions.

The intensity of a workout will determine the results received from the exercise. As one becomes stronger and in better shape, one will be able to increase the intensity of the workout and increase his progress.

MONITORING INTENSITY
(Record Keeping)

Keep track of the amount of time it takes to complete a workout, while also keeping a record of the number of sets and the amount of weight used for each exercise. In weight training, try to increase gradually the amount of weight that can be properly executed in a given exercise, while maintaining proper form.

Decrease the amount of time it takes for the total workout. This is accomplished by decreasing the amount of time between sets (resting time) to as little as one minute, not by decreasing the number of repetitions or exercises.

In aerobics, time and the amount of body activity generally govern intensity. The concept of aerobics is to condition the body's most important muscle, the heart, and to improve the operation of the cardiovascular system. The body must process oxygen efficiently, in order to facilitate the burning of nutrients as fuel for the muscles.

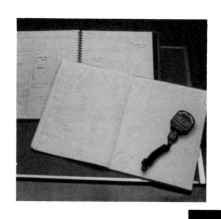

*P*roper aerobic activity raises the heart rate into the target zone (calculated as 220 minus your age, X .70) and maintains the target rate for at least 20 minutes, a minimum of three times a week. In aerobics classes, time usually remains finite, while the pace and workload increase.

*I*f running is your selected aerobic activity, either time or distance may be the fixed dimension. Say 20 minutes is the length of your run. You will find that as you become more fit, the distance you cover in a 20-minute period will increase, and thus, the run has become more intense. You have done more work in the same amount of time. A stronger heart can take on the heavier workload.

*I*f the distance is fixed, say at five miles, gradually decrease the length of time taken on course to increase intensity. A third variation might be to run part of the course uphill.

*T*rying a little harder, going a little further than the last time out, putting in the extra effort, just a little more than is comfortable, this is what will make the difference in results.

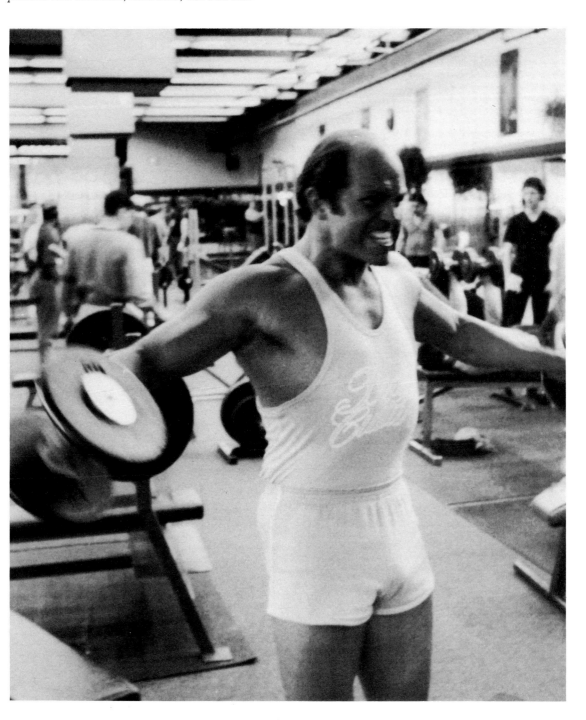

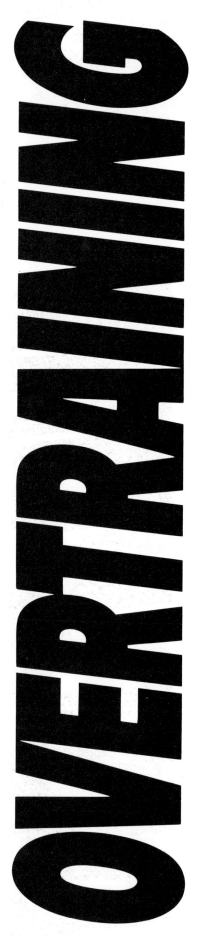

OVERTRAINING

For years, I thought that overtraining meant to train a part of the body too hard, or for too long a period of time on each workout.

These are not the problems, for you may train hard, and for long periods of time, often in a one-week period if you get sufficient rest for the body to recuperate and regenerate before it is worked again.

Overtraining would be understood more readily if it were referred to as "under-resting".

Often, an overly zealous trainee, in pursuit of superior fitness, feels that rest time is for softies. If one workout a day is good, then two are better; and so he increases the number of workouts to the point where recuperation is impossible. He keeps proceeding to another workout before the body has fully recovered from the previous workout.

This is particularly true of beginners. Because their ability to recover is much slower than that of a conditioned person, beginners need more time between workouts for best results.

Beginners should allow 48 to 60 hours between workouts. Here is a model for the first month of training:

1st week	Monday	Thursday	Sunday
2nd week	Wednesday	Saturday	Tuesday
3rd week	Friday	Monday	Thursday
4th week	Sunday	Wednesday	Saturday

This schedule allows plenty of time for recovery. For those taking on a full body weight training program or aerobics class, a regular weekly program for the next month could work well on Monday-Wednesday-Friday or Tuesday-Thursday-Saturday. This still allows 48 hours between workouts.

Eventually, you can work up to daily routines. Exercise every day if you desire, but don't repeat the same routine on consecutive days and don't stress the same body part (in weight training) two days in a row.

The exception to this would be aerobics for endurance. You can work up to daily sessions of aerobics exercises or running or swimming. This will greatly help to increase your endurance, but there must be some days of rest in the schedule. Even a veteran can suffer from overtraining.

WARNING SIGNS OF OVERTRAINING

1. The most common symptom is tiredness and lack of energy for your workout. It is both physical and psychological. Your ambition dwindles, and you can't get enthused about working out.

2. People say you look beat and ask if you are okay. They notice a drawn-out appearance, bags under your eyes, poor posture and lack of pizzazz.

3. The progress of your training either reaches a plateau or starts to reverse.

4. An increased susceptibility to injury due to diminished power or reflexes. Your tiredness affects concentration and makes you less coordinated.

5. Continuous muscle soreness and stiffness, because the muscles are not recuperating.

6. Poor performance in competition.
If you are suffering from the above symptoms, even though you may deny them to yourself, you cannot perform at your optimum.

7. Irritability is also a symptom of overtraining: over-reacting to the slightest problematic situation; showing poor sportsmanship; difficulties in interpersonal relationships.

The three most important components of physical fitness are exercise to work and develop the muscles; nutrition to feed the body and to provide energy and building materials; rest to allow the muscles to recover, and to build and increase in strength and stamina.

All of these components must receive equal attention. If any one of them is neglected, your results will suffer.

DISCIPLINE

Definition: training, especially of the mind or character; the training effect of experience; a trained condition of order and obedience; to bring under control.

The discipline necessary to accomplish good results from your exercise requires that training be consistent and persistent. Exercising only once a month does not bring results. A training program, once established, must be adhered to – with no excuses. If your program calls for three workouts a week, then three it is. A missed workout must be made up the same week.

Too often, we feel we have "reasons" for not working out that are really nothing more than excuses. We say there's no time, or that we're overworked or that we've had a hard day, or that the kids have drained us.

Counter these "reasons" by being unreasonable with yourself. It's your health that's at stake.

When I see a person who is obviously overweight, I visualize 20 or 30 pounds of excuses, alibis and reasons for the excess. They may be justifiable and very real, but the extra weight is just as real. Results are what counts.

People who are out of shape claim they don't have the time to work out, but neither do the people who are in shape. You have to make the time. Certainly there are duties associated with business, creative pursuits or family. Fitness is your duty too – a duty to yourself! And it is not just another labor, but a break from all the others, an outlet.

You must set your long-term objectives in health and fitness and make a commitment to them. Make the time. Be enthusiastic about yourself. You deserve the priority status you've been affording everyone and everything else.

I have found an excellent technique to make the time necessary for my workouts. In my personal appointment book, where I keep track of my daily business, I mark in workouts as meetings.

If someone were to ask for that time and I tell them I'm working out, there's a tendency for them to think of a workout as something unimportant, that can be skipped. Calling it a meeting puts it on the level of being official and important – and why shouldn't it be? Keep these appointments with yourself, consistently and persistently.

One weekend a month, I go to Montreal for a post-graduate course, and, rather than miss a workout, I double up the part of my routine that would be missed and do it on the Tuesday or Thursday of the week that I am away. While I'm in Montreal, I perform some other activity, such as playing squash or skiing, or do some exercise in my hotel room. It doesn't replace the workout, but it maintains the continuity of a physical program.

Continuity is important to stave off the effects of aging. It seems when you're in your twenties and naturally more active, you can miss weeks of working out and not notice much effect from the layoff, other than day-after soreness. In your thirties, a missed week can result in a couple of extra pounds of baggage and a decrease in strength, flexibility and endurance. In your forties and beyond, if your muscles aren't utilized and stretched regularly, they contract and shorten.

You may hit a plateau in your training where you do not feel progress. Your body has adapted to the type of workout your are doing there is no need for it to improve. This is the time to shock the system. Incorporate different exercises, change the amount of aerobic or weight training component in your program; use different workout equipment and change the pace.

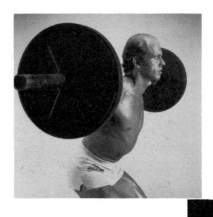

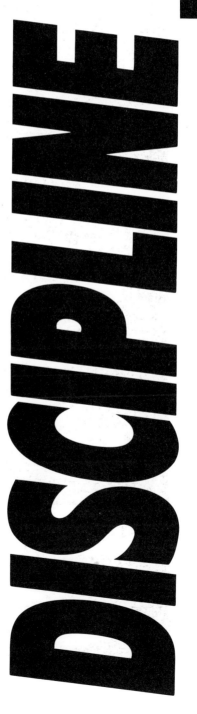

DISCIPLINE

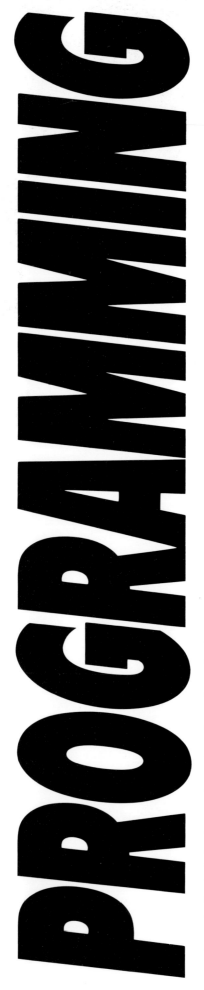

PROGRAMMING

PUTTING IT TOGETHER

Before putting your program together, get acquainted with some of the common terms in weight training and the various methods of performing and combining the exercises. I have arranged the terms in a gradient order, from beginners to advanced.

1. ROUTINE or program is the complete collection of exercises done for the entire body, usually in a one-week period.

2. REPETITION, abbreviated as Rep. is the complete execution of a particular exercise from start to finish, through its full range of motion.

3. SET is a series of consecutive repetitions, with little or no time interval between them. A set may consist of two to 20 repetitions. After a short rest, the next group of repetitions or set is performed.

4. REST between sets. Generally, beginners will take a longer pause to recuperate between sets. As one becomes more advanced, this rest time is shortened because the recuperative abilities improve. Beginners may take three to five minutes to get ready for the next set, while advanced trainers may be ready in as little as 10 seconds. Consciously decreasing this interval increases the intensity of the workout.

5. INTENSITY is the amount of effort exerted in performing an exercise. Intensity can be increased by adding weight, increasing repetitions, shortening the rest intervals, or by working to muscle failure of a particular muscle group. Intensity is also a psychological phenomenon, governing the effort expended. Most tests indicate maximum effort is only possible for advanced trainees but I have watched many beginners giving as much as possible.
That's what counts. The ability to train with increasing intensity does come with experience. Strive for it. The difference in results is dramatic!

6. CONCENTRATION is related to instensity. It is comical to watch some people merely going through the motions in the gym. I recall one day watching a very overweight member of a fitness club doing what were supposed to be torso twists. The only parts twisting were his ankles and arms. He was going through the motions, getting no benefit at all from his effort.

In weight training, allowing a weight to drop, instead of lowering it or swinging the weight to get momentum does not entitle you to results. The exercise must be performed under complete control.
This is done through concentration and vizualization. Concentrate on the particular muscle being worked. See it working. Vizualize it shortening, contracting to move the weight in the direction you desire. Vizualize it getting bigger, stronger. Do this with each rep. This ability alone will increase the specificity of isolation and complete contraction to maximize results.
To improve your ability to vizualize muscles in various body parts, we have included anatomical sketches in the weight training section.
When someone tells me he gets bored doing a certain exercise, that reveals he is not concentrating. If you are thinking of other things, you cannot concentrate. Don't talk to anyone when he is performing an exercise. Let him concentrate.

7. PROGRESSION in resistance on the muscles is the key to weight training. The body will adapt to the stresses by growing or stretching or becoming more fit in a cardiovascular sense. Once the body has adapted, if the stress is not progressively increased, the improvement slows to a stop. By progressively increasing the intensity of the workouts, the body is continually forced to adapt further.

8. RECORD KEEPING is necessary to keep track of your progress. By writing down the weights, reps, sets and any comments on each workout, you have an accurate reference point from which to start the next session and can appropriately increase the intensity.
Keeping records allows your mind the freedom to concentrate on performing the exercise and isolating the muscles rather than trying to remember what you did last time.
Occasionally measure and weight yourself to check on your progress and record these figures in the exercise log as well. Take pictures every six months to see the gradual transformation and the effects of your dedication.

BEGINNERS

The novice who jumps right into a heavy, intensive workout often injures himself and usually can hardly walk or move his parts well for a week. The pain may be so bad that he is totally discouraged and may never work out again.

It takes time to get in shape. For the beginner, it takes two to three weeks of initial training to get in good enough shape for a good workout. Then, the real training starts. The body must first get accustomed to the movements and the weights to be used. It will require some experimenting to determine the correct poundage for each exercise.

The beginners' program consists of doing very basic exercises for each workout, emphasizing correct form as described in the text. For best results, work the large muscle groups first, because you have the most energy at the start of the work-out. If you work the small muscles to exhaustion first, there won't be enough energy left to work the larger groups sufficiently to stimulate change.

Exercises should be arranged in the following order:
1. legs; 2. back; 3. shoulders; 4. chest; 5. triceps; 6. biceps; 7. calfs; 8. forearms; 9. abdominals.

ROUTINE 1

Beginners' exercises, in proper order:
1. Warm up
2. Squats
3. Bent-over rowing
4. Standing shoulder press
5. Bench press
6. Tricep extensions
7. Barbell curls
8. Calf raise
9. Wrist curls
10. Abdominal Crunch
11. Stretch for each part of the body.

The scheduling for this program should allow 48 to 60 hours between workouts, to permit sufficient recuperation time.

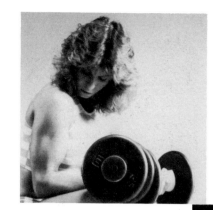

SETS AND REPETITIONS

First Month

Do one set of each exercise, choosing a weight that allows you to complete only 10 to 12 repetitions. Exceptions are the calf, forearms and legs, where 20 repetitions may be attained, and the abdominals, which should be given as many reps as possible. The rest time for a beginning workout is abou three minutes. The total workout time for the beginner is about 52 minutes: 10 minutes to warm up, 37 minutes to complete nine exercises (plus rest) and a five-minute stretch session at the end.
Note: Add weight in each exercise when you can do more than the prescribed number of reps.

Second Month

Once the beginner's routine is comfortable, increase to two sets of each exercise. Consciously start to decrease the length of rest time between exercises to two minutes and you will be able to keep the workout to about an hour. You are increasing the intensity of the workout.

Third Month

Increase to three sets of each exercise, still doing the basic exercises. Add weights as you get stronger and continue to decrease the rest periods to one minute.

After three months of basic exercises, you will have seen general progress in all areas of your physique. Now you are ready to start experimenting with other types of exercises, to see which ones your body best responds to. Everyone is different and some exercises work better for some than for others.

Those who are more fit will be able to progress from one set to two and three sets in a short time period. If you can, fine. But stick to the basic exercises for three months. Doing so ensures a sound basis for greater progress later.

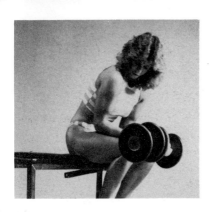

INTERMEDIATE

At the intermediate level, you should be confident in your ability to monitor your reactions to the different exercises and ready to introduce some variety, all the while increasing intensity.

Some new training principles can be introduced at this stage:

1. MUSCLE FAILURE in weight training is achieved at the end of a set, when a maximum effort fails to move the weight any more, without assistance. If you can still do a partial repetition, continue to failure. Performing those numbers of reps which are comfortable will only maintain the muscular development you've achieved. Further improvement requires more effort.
I do not believe in the philosophy of "No pain, no gain." I do believe in more effort, more gain. Sometimes, pain is an indication that something is wrong. Pay attention to the body's warning signals. A burning feeling in the muscles is common and temporary. It is usually relieved upon finishing the set and stretching. If not, have it checked out.

2. FORCED REPS can be done after failure is reached, with the assistance of your training partner. His aid is minimal, just enough to get the weight past the difficult point. This allows you to perform two or three more reps you couldn't otherwise do, at the end of the set. This technique is recommended for areas that need extra attention, not for every exercise.

3. CHEATING is used to make the completion of a set harder, not easier. It is a method of doing forced reps when no training partner is available. Once you reach the failure point in an exercise, slightly swing the weight and recruit other muscle groups for assistance. For example, in the standing press, a slight upward thrust with the legs may be used to start the weight in motion.
Cheating does not reflect proper form, and is not to be used before failure sets in. Like forced reps, it is not to be over-utilized.

4. NEGATIVE phase of an exercise describes the lowering of the weight to starting position. This part of the exercise increases the potential for improvement by taking the muscle through its full range of motion, using a greater percentage of the muscle fibres in the group. Negative emphasis is a technique in which the negative phase of the exercise is slowed down and performed under complete control.
In assisted negatives, your partner raises the weight to the up position and you lower it through the negative phase, as slowly as possible.

5. PRIORITY TRAINING is the process of placing exercise emphasis on weak spots or parts of the body that aren't responding as well as others. Genetically, we aren't given perfectly symmetrical physiques and a look in the mirror confirms this. Simply train those weaker parts of the body harder, longer and more often. Do the area needing the most work at the start of the workout, when the energy level is at its highest.

6. STICKING POINTS. Progress is slow but steady in most cases. Occasionally, one or more body parts refuses to progress with the rest of the body, even though it is worked as intesively as all the rest. If this persists more than a few weeks, the muscles are becoming accustomed to a particular type of training and have adapted comfortably to the stresses applied. They do not need to progress any more.
One solution is to take a week off from weight training, to rest the body. Do other athletic activities, but take a holiday from weights. Just as when you take a break from school or work, you enthusiasm is rekindled and refreshed when you come back. Return to a totally new routine, changing the exercises, the order, the sets and the reps. Keep it interesting.

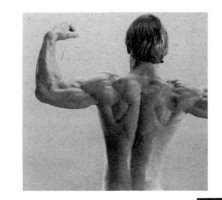

ROUTINES FOR INTERMEDIATES

At this point, you are ready to introduce more than one exercise per body part. The following routines use exercises from the weight training section.

ROUTINE 2

Warm up	10 minutes (see warm up section).
Abdominals	full leg raises, 6-inch leg raise, oblique crunch, upper crunch.
Legs	lunge, Jefferson squat.
Back	chins, single rowing.
Shoulders	upright rowing, flies.
Chest	incline press, dumbell flies.
Triceps	French press, dips.
Biceps	alternating curls, concentration curls.
Calfs	sitting raise, donkeys.
Forearms	reverse curl, barbell behind back wrist curl.

Sets and Reps – For abdominals, do one set of each exercise, as many repetitions as possible. For all the rest, except calfs and forearms, do six to eight reps for building muscle mass, 10 to 12 reps for shaping. Start applying the training principles of failure, forced reps, cheating, negative emphasis and priority training to the intermediate routine.
Do the above routine for two months, starting with two sets of each. Then you work up to three sets.

ROUTINE 3

Warm up	10 to 15 minutes of aerobics and stretching.
Abdominals	full program of six exercises and twists.
Legs	hack squats, lunge.
Back	bent-over rowing, hyperextensions.
Shoulders	dumbell shoulder press, shrugs.
Chest	decline press, pull over.
Triceps	one-arm extention, kick backs.
Biceps	dumbell curl sitting, incline curls.
Calfs	single dumbell raise, dumbell sitting raise.
Forearms	wrist curl dumbell, reverse wrist curl barbell.

Do the routine for two months, increasing intensity as before. Again, with the exception of the abdominals, do two sets of each and progress to three sets as soon as possible.

ADVANCED

By now, your workouts are starting to get lengthy because of the number of exercises in the routine. It is time for you to break up the workout, doing different body parts on separate days. Notice, however, that abdomonal exercises may be done at each workout. We follow with an example of a three-day split. In this routine, you would do the full abdominal program, changing it from time to time with some of the abdominal exercises from the aerobics section. For each body part, do three different exercises, and for stubborn body parts, you may wish to do more exercises or more than three sets. Include the basic exercises from the beginning stage and blend them with exercises from intermediate and advanced stages.

ROUTINE 4

Monday	Abdominals	six exercises and twists
	Legs	squat, lunge, Jefferson squat
	Calfs	barbell calf raise, donkeys, singles
	Shoulders	standing press, upright rowing, flies
Wednesday	Abdominals	same routine
	Chest	bench & decline presses, barrel flies.
	Back	dead lift, chins, single rowing.
Friday	Abdominals	same routine
	Triceps	extensions, kick backs, French press
	Biceps	barbell curls, alternate curls, concentration curls.
	Forearms	reverse curls, wrist curls, behind the back barbell curls.

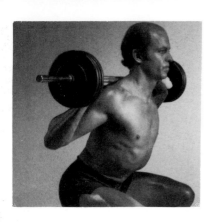

We can now also introduce the last series of terms and techniques to provide increased intensity and variety in the workout.

1. SUPER SETS are done when two different exercises are performed, one right after the other, with little or no rest between. Usually, opposing muscle groups are involved.
For example, you can pair bicep-tricep (bicep curl and tricep press), or chest-back (bench press and bent-over rowing), or stomach-back (abdominal crunches and hyperextensions). Super sets may also be used for different parts of the same major muscles. The incline bench press, which works the upper pectorals, can be super setted with the decline bench press for the lower and outer pectorals. Chins, for the upper back, can be super setted with dead lifts for the lower back and lats.

2. TRI SETS are a method of incorporating three different exercises together for one body part with little or no rest between the exercises. This greatly increases the intensity of the workout.
For example, a chest tri set could consist of the bench press, followed by the incline press and barrel flies. A back tri set could involve the dead lift, bent-over rowing and hyperextensions. The shoulder tri set uses the front, side and rear lateral raise exercises.

3. GIANT SETS are done by combining four to six different exercises together in close succession, with little or no rest between sets. A giant set for the chest may consist of bench press, incline press, decline press and barrel flies. A giant set for the back might include the dead lift, bent-over-rowing, single rowing and hyperextensions.
Giant sets are more intensive than super sets or tri sets and are hard on the body. They are not to be done as a regular routine, except for the abdominal program, which may be done as a giant set.

4. PEAK CONTRACTION. The more muscles that are utilized in an exercise, the better the progress. This is done by contracting the muscle fully at the top, or peak of the exercise and keeping weight resistance on it at that point. You may want to alter the angle of the exercise, so that there is no static rest point at the top of the movement, where the muscle doesn't bear any weight. At the top of the move, squeeze and hold for a full second or more.

5. STRIPPING is another method of continuing past failure. When you cannot do another rep, either switch to a lighter dumbell or have your training partner quickly strip off some weight. Continue to failure again, then remove more weight, until you have stripped down to the bar only. You will feel a burning sensation in the muscle. This is from a buildup of lactic acid and is normal.

6. DOWN THE RACK is another method similar to stripping, using a full rack of dumbells. Do a single exercise, such as standing curls, staring with the heaviest weight your can handle, changing to the next lightest set of dumbells when you hit muscle failure, with no rest between weights. Stripping and down the rack are very intense routines and should only be done once or twice a month for each body part.

7. REST PAUSE. When lifting heavy weights, the muscles gradually build up fatigue toxins and oxygen stores are depleted. This limits the number of reps that can be done before failure. By pausing for a few deep breaths at the point of failure, the body can eliminate some of the toxins and get some oxygen to the muscle, allowing you to do two or three more reps. Then pause again. Rest 10 to 15 seconds and do as many more reps as you can. Rest pause training is very intense and should only be done by an advanced trainer.

8. CIRCUIT TRAINING can actually be used at any level to increase the cardiovascular endurance and to burn off excess fat. It consists of performing a series of 10 to 20 exercises, one after the other, without rest. For example, the beginner's routine can be done with little or no rest between sets. Then take a rest of two to four minutes and start again, without the warm up.

The goal is to decrease the time it takes you to do a circuit, while maintaining the poundage for the exercise. A circuit of nine exercises could take as little as nine minutes to perform. Initially, the routine is exhausting, but with practice it will increase your endurance and general fitness level. You can work up to three or four circuits in a hour.

9. POSING is the art of displaying your physique and is an excellent workout in itself. Practice in front of a mirror, flexing the various muscle groups. You will become quite proficient at it and will never have an excuse not to exercise. You can pose anywhere, without equipment.

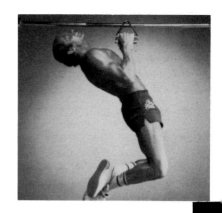

Contract and hold the muscle in a flexed position, as hard as you can for 10 seconds. This is an excellent way to improve your control over your muscles and to improve the cuts and lines in muscle definition. A mirror is a must as part of your exercise equipment, to judge progress and form.

CONCLUSION

It becomes apparent that to maximize your potential for muscle stength and size, you must implement a wide variety of techniques. Use light and heavy weights, high and low numbers of repetitions, positive and negative phases of exercises. Experiment and see what works best for your various body parts. Be persistent and consistent with the workouts. Keep changing, keep learning and keep improving.

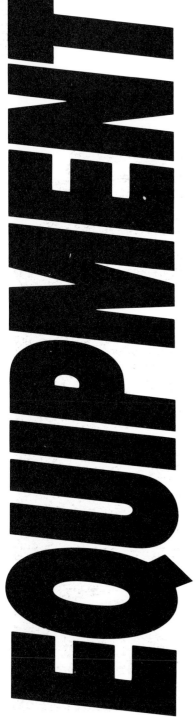

EQUIPMENT

The equipment selected for the exercises in the weight training section is very simple. It can be purchased for a modest amount and used in the home. Should you have access to gym facilities, the exercises are adaptable to the various types of equipment there.

Barbell: consists of a long steel bar, varying in length from four feet to seven feet, with or without a sleeve, weight plates and collars to hold the weights in place.

Dumbell: a one-hand version of the barbell, 10 to 14 inches long and having the same component parts. Dumbells are usually used in matched pairs, one in each hand.

Bench: should be adjustable to allow for supine and incline positions during exercises.

Safety Racks: an important feature for such exercises as squats and bench press, made of cast iron, with a large metal base, an upright adjustable post and resting "catch" for the barbell.

Wood Block: three pieces of 2 x 12-inch pine, two feet long, nailed together, to be used as a calf block, dead lift block and decline block for the bench.

Chiro Grips: Foam grips to improve your grip and help prevent callouses.

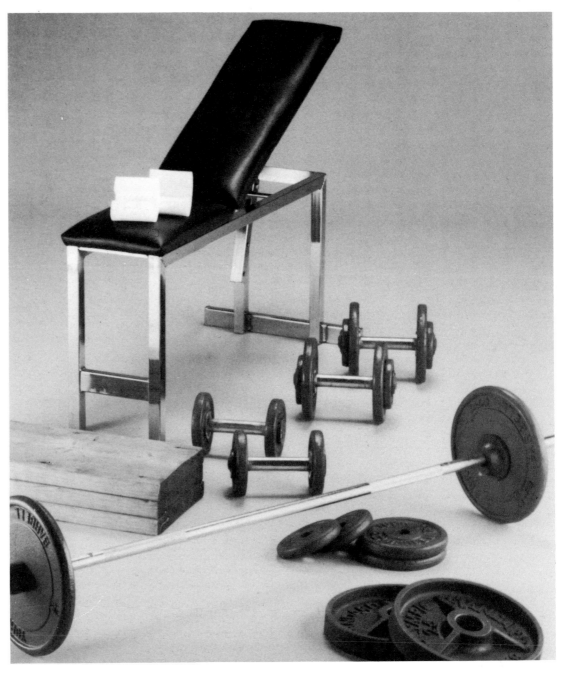

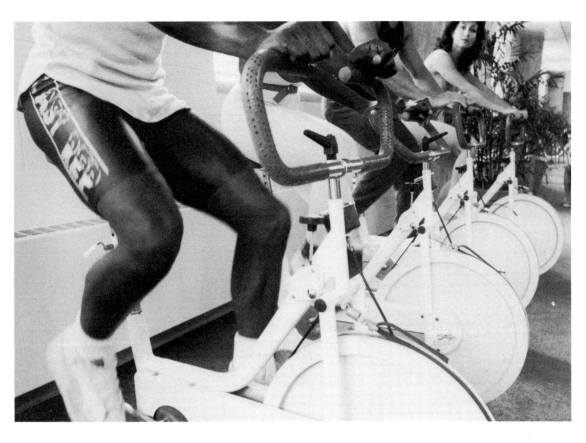

WARM UP

A cold muscle does not stretch or contract well and is susceptible to injury. The same applies to the connective tissue, the ligaments and tendons. Warming up means increasing the circulation generally, and particularly to the parts of the body to be exercised.

A simple comparison experiment demonstrates the necessity of a warm up. Perform your routine one day, without a warm up. Note your strength accomplishment, degree of endurance, flexibility and muscle soreness. Do the same workout on another day with a proper warm up and make the same follow-up observations.

The differences will be measureable. Not only will the performance be better, but there will be more energy and less muscle soreness. These factors greatly decrease the incidence of injury. The warm up increases the heart rate and speeds up circulation, augmented by an increase in respiration, bringing oxygen to the muscles. The warm, supple muscles stretch better, allowing a breater range of motion in the performance of exercises.

Professional athletes know an extensive warm up improves the ability to perform and to co-ordinate the movements required for their sports.

FORMAT

Begin the workout with five minutes of mild aerobic exercise, such as riding a stationary bike at low tension, jumping rope, stride jumps or jogging.

Adjust the bike seat high enough to allow the outstretched leg to extend almost fully and pedal at a moderate speed. Note: If you want a cardiovascular training effect, a ride of at least 20 minutes with the heart working at 75 per cent of maximum capacity is necessary.

Proceed to general stretches, beginning with the larger, load-bearing muscles of the legs. Check the form for all the stretches: hamstring stretch; calf stretch; quad stretch; chest stretch; shoulder stretch; back stretch.

For the next part of the warm up, I perform my abdominal routine, using exercises for each of the four diferent sections of the abdominal muscles – upper, middle, lower and oblique. After the abdominals get the blood pumping, go on to stretches for specific muscles prior to exercising each body part. Finally, start each set of the workout using a very light weight, and concentrate on a grooved form. Perform 15 to 20 reps at a medium speed, under great control to get the muscles warm and ready for the intensity and effort of your workout.

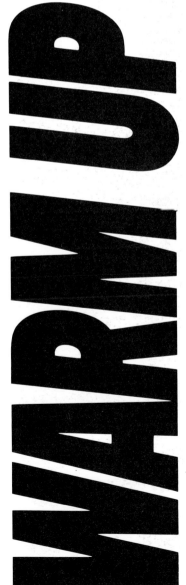

WARM UP

ABDOMINALS

Strong abdominal muscles are helpful in almost every activity. They maintain erect posture and are the major supporting structure for the back. The abdominals must also shield the internal organs of the mid-section.

Many people are of the opinion that abdominal exercises will get rid of the excess fat on the waistline. This is not the case. Spot fat reducing is not possible, for exercise of any kind uses up calories which are taken evenly from the fat stores of the body.

To reduce the fat content of the abdomen, you must reduce the fat content of the entire body. To do this, take fewer calories into the body in the way of food and burn more calories through exercise. The exercises will increase the musculature for a firmer, trimmer figure. Many large abdominal areas are more than just fat deposits. If you were to examine the fat content under the skin, you would find one or two inches of fat, but not enough to account for some large pot bellies. What you are observing is the result of a slow or stagnant digestive system (colon). A build-up of partially digested food can lodge in the intestines and is frequently associated with constipation. This can be an accumulation of five to 20 pounds in some cases!

A thorough cleansing may be necessary. Colonic irrigation is the fastest method and many herbal cleansers are available to help eliminate this potentially dangerous and toxic accumulation.

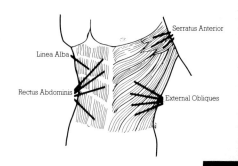

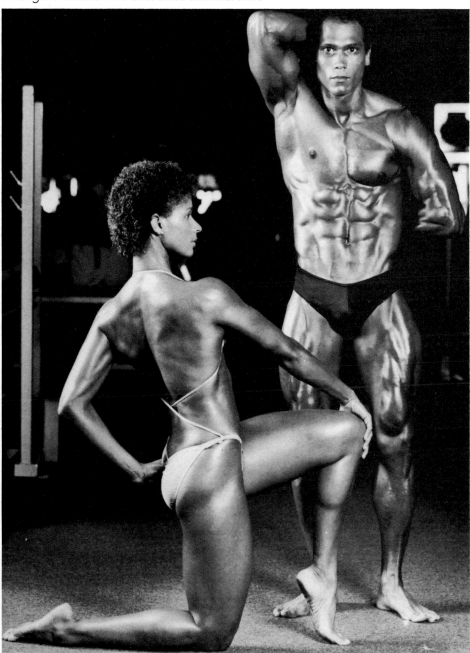

Photo: Chris Lund

LEG RAISE

Muscle Group:
Lower abdominals.

Position:
Sit on the end of the bench, grasp the end of the bench with your hands under your buttocks. Lean back far enough to outstretch the legs and have the body in a straight line. Do not touch the floor.

Form:
Raise your legs up as high as possible by contrtacting the stomach muscles only. Also, flex the neck forward for a complete abdominal contraction. Hold for one second, then slowly release.

KNEE TO FOREHEAD

Muscle Group:
Lower abdominals.

Position:
Sit on the end of the bench, with hands and legs in same position as for the leg raise.

Form:
With knees slightly bent, pull the legs up using only the abdominals and flex the head forward to have the knee touch the forehead. Fully flex the abdominals at the top position and hold for one second, then slowly release.

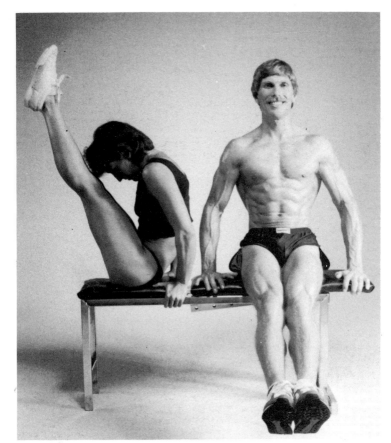

LEG RAISE

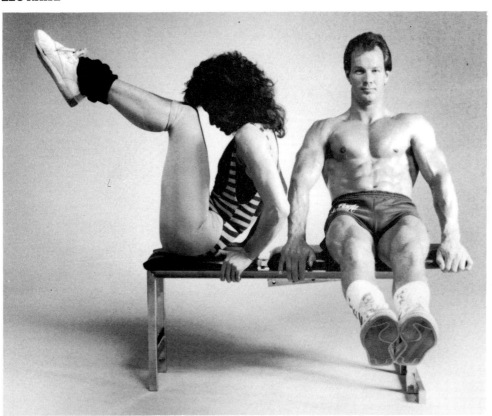

KNEE TO FOREHEAD

SIX-INCH LEG RAISES

Muscle Group:
Lower abdmoninals.

Position:
Lie supine (face up) on the floor, with the hands palms down under your buttocks.
Raise the feet to 6 inches off the floor.

Form:
Bring the feet to only 12 inches from the floor, using the lower abdominals, and pull the chin toward your chest at the same time.

Pointer:
Concentrate on using the lower abdominals only. This will take a little practice, as most of us are used to using the psoas to do this exercise. If this exercise is done incorrectly and the major muscle used is the psoas, it can irritate existing low back problems.

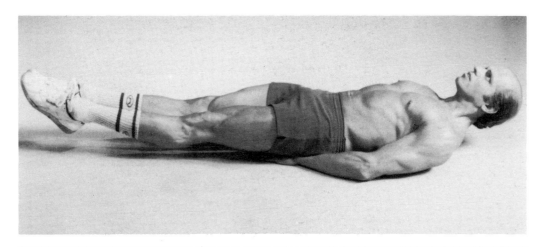

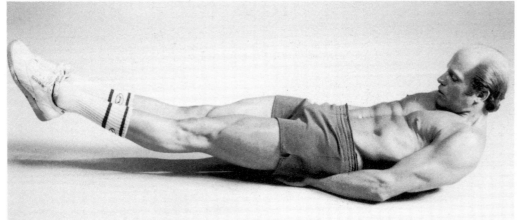

CROSS CRUNCH

Muscle Groups:
Obliques and right and left rectus abdominals. This will increase the definition of the mid-line split (aderncrosis) between the rectus abdominus.

Position:
Lie supine on the floor, legs bent and feet flat on the floor. The hands touch the temples and the elbows are flared out.

Form:
Slowly raise your head and start curling the right shoulder toward the left knee, crunching as hard as possible and also flexing the right hip at the same time. Touch the right elbow to the left knee. Hold for one second, then lower to starting position. Repeat by curling the left shoulder toward the right knee and flexing the left hip. Hold and lower.

Pointer:
Feel the abdominal muscles working on one side at a time.

FRONT CRUNCH

Muscle Group:
Upper middle rectus abdominus.

Position:
Lie supine on the floor, hands at your side, knees bent.

Form:
Raise the head and shoulders and curl them toward the knees as far as possible, reaching with your outstretched hands toward the feet. The pelvis is tilted up and toward the head. Pull in as hard as possible and flex. Hold for two seconds. Release and repeat.

Pointer:
Do not raise the pelvis off the ground. Make sure you are crunching hard enough and holding long enough and are not resting too long in the down position. Contract and squeeze the area as hard as possible. Having the arms outstretched assists this.

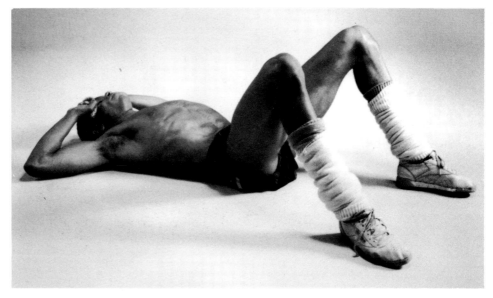

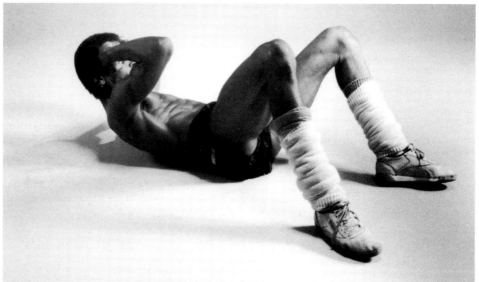

CROSS CRUNCH

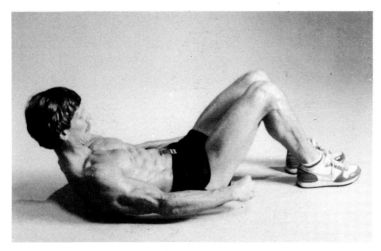

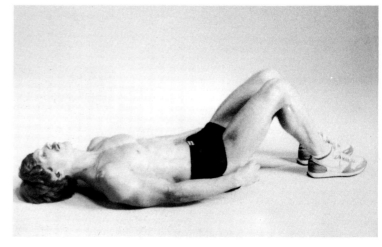

FRONT CRUNCH

HEAD RAISE

Muscle Group:
Uppermost rectus abdominus.

Position:
Lie supine on the floor, calves resting on top of the bench and elbows flared out with the hands on the temples.

Form:
Lift your head and shoulders toward the ceiling and lower to the starting position. Concentrate on squeezing the upper abdominals.

Pointer:
Rest the legs; they are not involved in this exercise. Lift the upper body, do not curl.

TWISTS

Muscle Groups:
Internal and external obliques, with secondary stress on the lower back.

Equipment:
Unweighted bar or broomstick.

Position:
Stand with the feet six to eight inches wider than shoulder width apart. Place the bar behind neck, across the shoulders, holding the bar with the wrists, rather than fingers. Bend the knees slightly.

Form:
Twist in one direction as far as possible, then to the other. Do 50 full twists, then do shorter radius turns, forcibly stopping the rapid movement before the complete twist. Do 50 repetitions. This uses the obliques even more intensively than full twists.

Pointer:
If the knees are not bent, you get too much hip rotation, which decreases the effectiveness of the exercise.

Variations:
1. Sitting position eliminates hip movement.
2. You may twist your head as well or keep it facing forward for different stresses.

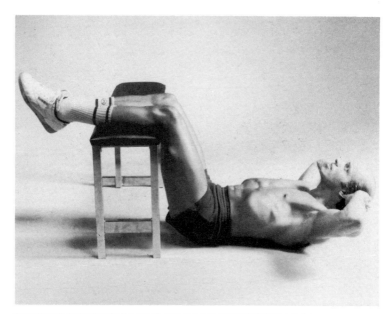

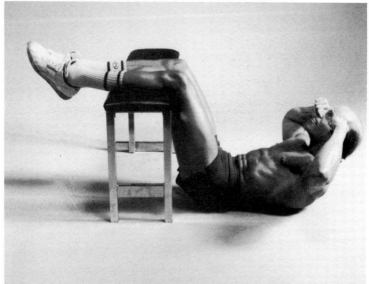

HEAD RAISE

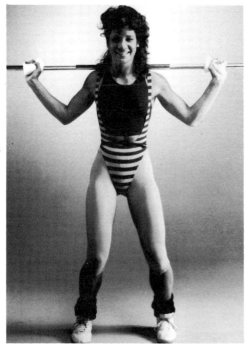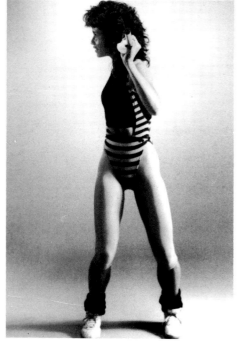

TWISTS

41

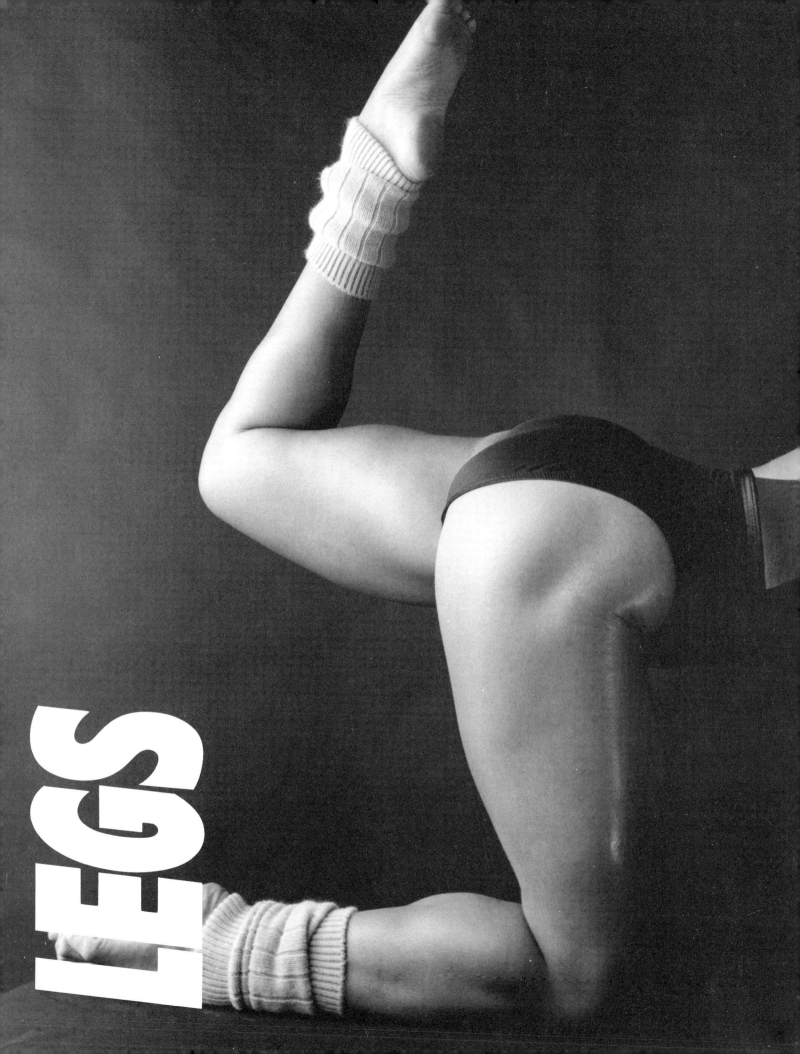

LEGS

BASIC SQUATS

Purpose:
1. To increase the strength of the quadriceps.
2. To increase the lung capacity.
3. To speed up the metabolism.

Muscle Group:
Quadriceps (front thighs).

Secondary Support Groups:
Hamstrings, lower and upper back, abdominals, buttocks, trapezius and calf. The heart and lungs benefit and there is increased circulation and metabolism.

Equipment:
1. Squat rack.
2. Barbell.
3. Weightlifting belt.

Position:
Lift the weight off the rack by placing the bar across the trapezius muscles. With a narrow hand grip, maintain this position (a close hand grip contracts the trapezius and gives a better cushion for the bar to rest upon). Feet are shoulder width apart, angled out 30 to 45 degrees for stability. A board, one to two inches thick, may be used under the heels for those with tight Achilles tendons, who find it difficult to keep the heels on the floor. This will improve balance. A training partner or spotter should be standing behind the squatter, to aid in balance or to help the exerciser rise if he is stuck in the down position. Do warm-ups without weights or with the bar only.

Form:
Look straight ahead, head up. The back is straight. Slowly lower yourself by bending the knees forward, over the feet. Keep the back straight and use abdominal muscles to maintain balance. Continue down until the thighs are parallel to the floor. Rise to starting position by pushing with the legs. Be careful not to arch the back. Do not bounce at the bottom of the squat, as this can damage the knees. A slight forward lean is necessary to keep the center of gravity over the feet. Variations in stance will work different muscles. A narrow stance of eight to 12 inches works the outer thighs. A wide stance of 30 inches works the inner thighs. A medium stance of about 16 inches works the upper thighs.

Pointers:
1. Allowing the back to arch inward or to round over can cause lower back injury. A weightlifting belt adds to lower back stability.
2. Do the squat in front of a mirror to observe your form.
3. Keep tight. Your position on the way down will determine efficiency on the way up. With heavy weights, the knees tend to come together on the way up. Force them out to the side to help maintain form. Also have a training partner correct your form.
4. If you feel yourself leaning too far forward, lift your chin up as you come up. This helps maintain balance.

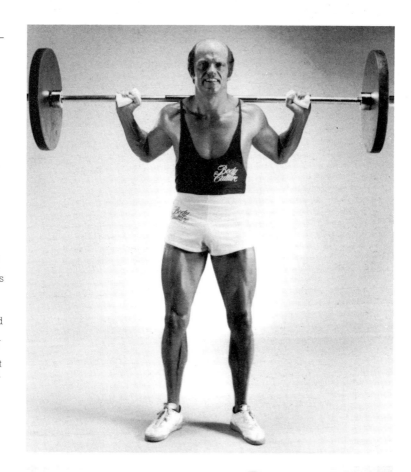

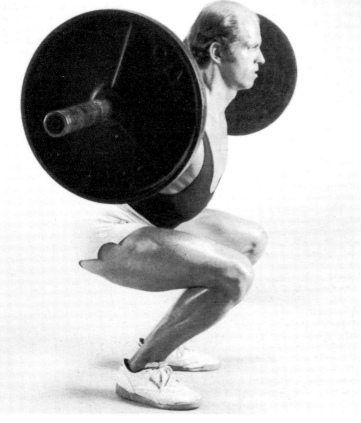

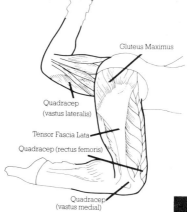

Gluteus Maximus
Quadracep (vastus lateralis)
Tensor Fascia Lata
Quadracep (rectus femoris)
Quadracep (vastus medial)

THE LUNGE

Muscle Groups:
Quadriceps femoris (front thighs), gluteus maximus (buttocks), biceps femoris, semitendinosis and semimembranosis (hamstring).

Equipment:
Barbell or dumbells.

Position:
Stand with barbell behind your head, across the trapezius muscles, or stand with dumbells at you side.

Form:
Keep the back straight and head up. Step forward with the left foot, 24 to 30 inches. Bend the left knee until the left thigh is parallel to the floor. Your right heel will come off the ground and the right knee will be close to the floor. Then push with the left leg back to staring position. Alternate legs.

Pointers:
A short step of two feet stresses the thigh muscles. A longer step stresses the buttocks. Men and especially women find this an excellent way to firm up these muscles.

HACK SQUAT

Muscle Group:
Quadriceps.

Secondary Support Groups:
Hamstrings and buttocks.

Equipment:
Barbell or dumbells.

Position:
Grip the bar behind you at arm's length, hands shoulder width apart or wider, palms facing back. The feet are shoulder width apart and the back is kept straight.

Form:
Slowly squat down until the thighs are almost parallel to the floor. The knees will flare slightly to the sides, in line with the feet. Face forward, head up, back straight. Return to starting position by straightening the legs.

Variations:
1. Narrower foot stance stresses the outer thigh.
2. When the hack squat is performed with dumbells, weights are held at the side. Follow the same form.
3. To stress the sartorius (inner thigh), the upper and the middle thigh, lift the weight as described in starting position, then assume a foot position slightly wider than shoulder width, with toes pointed out at 45 degrees. Keep the knees in line with the feet.

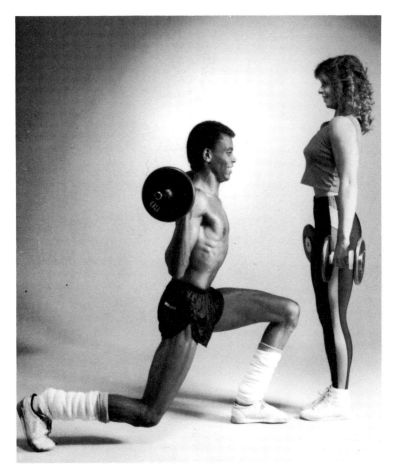

THE LUNGE

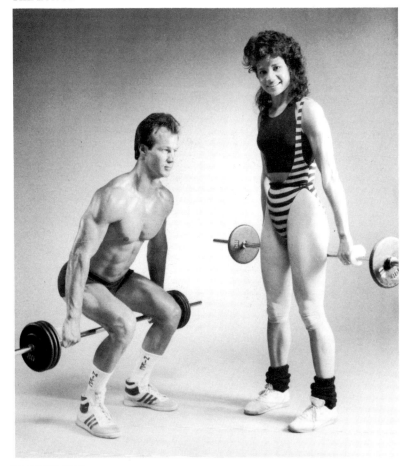

HACK SQUAT

JEFFERSON SQUAT

Muscle Groups:
Inner thighs, buttocks and lower back.

Equipment:
Barbell.

Position:
Straddle the barbell, with the feet 24 inches apart. Squat down and grasp the bar with one hand in front and the other behind, palms facing in. Keep the arms straight, back straight and head up.

Form:
Straighten the legs to full upright position, using the thighs, buttocks and lower back. Flex the thighs at the top position, hold. Lower the weight by bending the knees until the thighs are almost parallel to the floor.

Pointer:
Twist the bar sideways to permit the back to stay straight. Switch hands, front and back, on each set.

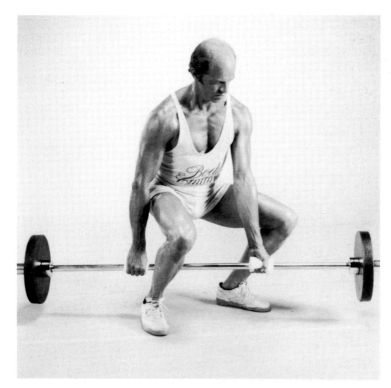

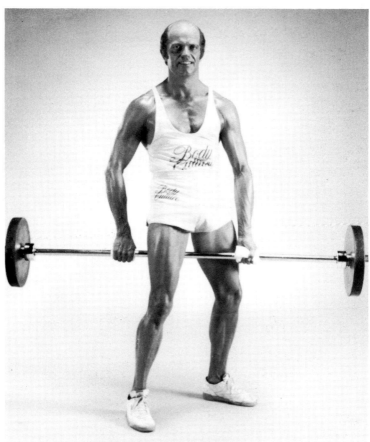

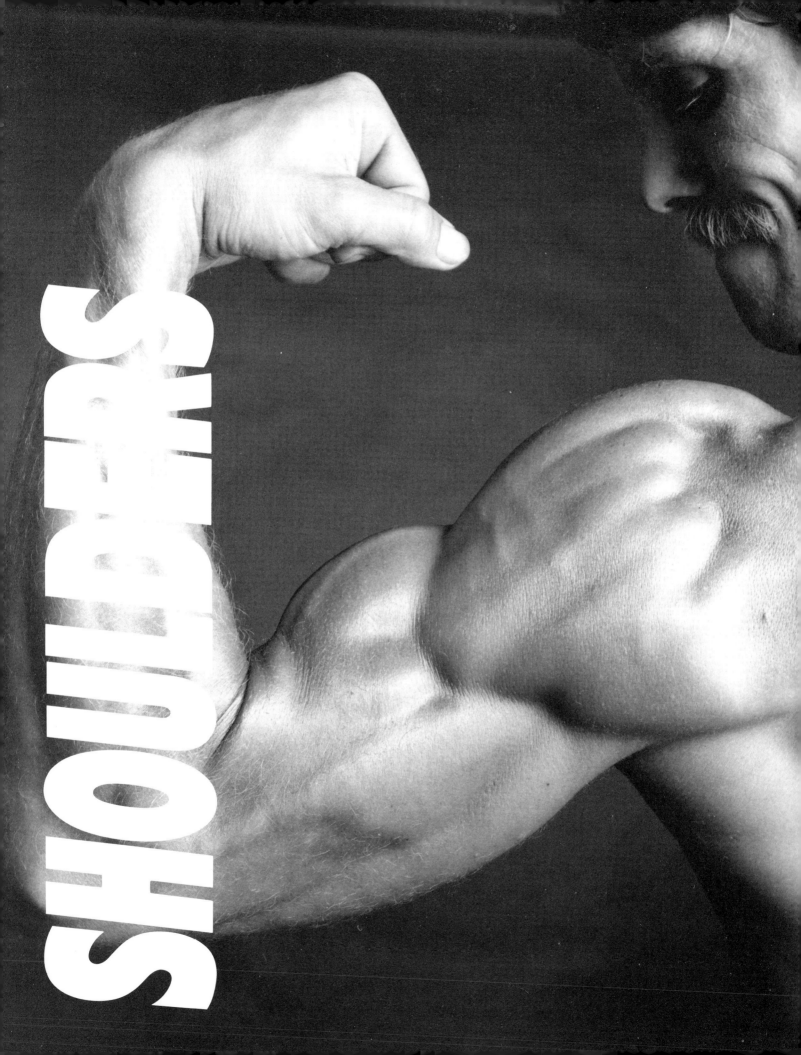

SHOULDERS

SHOULDER PRESS STANDING

Purpose:
To strengthen and develop the shoulders. This aids in overhead movements, pushing or reaching.

Muscle Group:
Anterior deltoid (more than military), triceps and trapezius.

Secondary Support Groups:
Upper pectoral muscles, serratus anterior.

Position:
Grip the bar two to four inches wider than shoulder width, palms facing forward. Pull the bar up to your chest and press it up over your head, lowering it behind the neck and resting it on the trapezius. Feet are shoulder width apart (one may be slightly forward for balance). Lock the legs and hips for stability. A spotter should be directly behind the person doing the lift. Assistance may be given in the last repetition or two by helping to push the elbows up.

Form:
Press the weight up to fully-extended arm's length. Lower slowly to touch trapezius, then repeat. Keep the back straight; avoid arching it. Do not use the legs to assist lifting the weight.

MILITARY PRESS

Muscle Groups:
Anterior deltoid, triceps, serratus anterior.

Secondary Support Groups:
Upper pectorals (more than standing press), trapezius.

Position:
Similar to standing press, but weight rests in front, on upper chest. Grip is shoulder width.

Form:
Press the bar up, just in front of face, to fully extended arm's lenth, and lower again to upper chest. Keep the elbows tucked closer than in standing press. This works the upper pectorals. Do not arch the back. The exercise can be performed in sitting position, to eliminate assistance from the legs.

NOT ILLUSTRATED

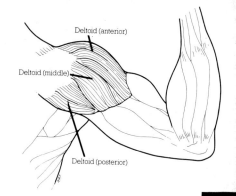

Deltoid (anterior)

Deltoid (middle)

Deltoid (posterior)

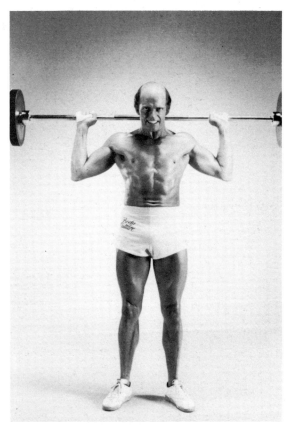

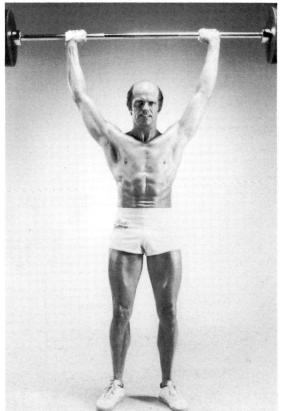

SHOULDER PRESS STANDING

THREE-WAY FLIES

Muscle Groups:
1. Front fly – Anterior deltoid and pectorals.
2. Side fly – Middle deltoid and trapezius.
3. Rear bent fly – Posterior deltoid, infras spinatus and teres.

Equipment:
Light dumbells.

Positions:
Front and side fly – Stand with feet shoulder width apart, arms at your sides, a dumbell in each hand.
Rear bent fly – Same position, but bend from the waist until upper body is parallel to the floor, with arms hanging down.

Form:
Front fly – Raise the dumbells slowly, palms down, arms straight in front of you until they are above shoulder height. Lower the weights, under control.
Side fly – Raise the dumbells to the side, with a straight arm, palms down, to above shoulder height. Hold and return.
Rear bent fly – Start in down position, palms facing each other. Bend the arms slightly, raise the arms up as far as possible, out to the side. Finish the move with the arms fully turned in (pronated), as though you were pouring something. This motion stresses the rear deltoid more than if the weight were lifted straight up with palms facing down.

Pointer:
Maintain complete control and do not swing the weight up.

Variation:
You may use the incline bench to reduce any body movement that would assist the shoulders.

Repetitions:
Do the three types of flies as a tri-set. Perform eight to 12 repetitions of each exercise, then rest two minutes and repeat the tri-set.

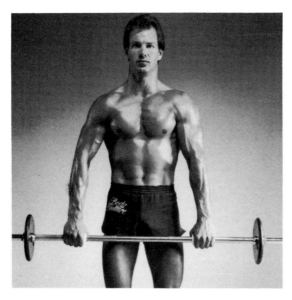
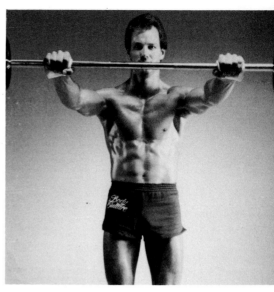
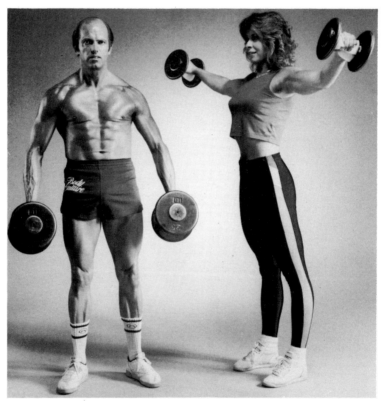
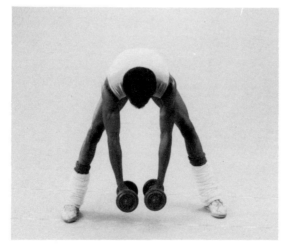
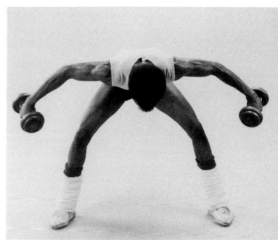

SHRUGS

Muscle Group:
Trapezius.

Equipment:
Heavy barbell.

Position:
Stand with your feet shoulder width apart. Grasp the barbell at shoulder width, palms facing you. Keep the arms straight and the bar resting against the upper thighs. Lower the shoulders slightly forward.

Form:
From the down position, raise (shrug) the shoulders up and slightly back in a semi-circular motion, as high as possible. Lower by reversing the motion back to the starting position.

Variations:
1. Do the semi-circular motion from back to front.
2. Raise the shoulders straight up and down.
3. Exercise may be done using a pair of dumbells together, or by working the shoulders alternately.

Pointer:
With a very heavy barbell, you may have the weight supported by the bench press rack at the start of the exercise.

UPRIGHT ROWING

Muscle Groups:
Anterior and middle deltoid, trapezius.

Secondary Support Groups:
Biceps, brachiordials, brachialis.

Equipment:
Barbell.

Position:
Stand with feet shoulder width apart. Grasp the bar with hands six to eight inches apart, palms facing you. Have the bar hang down in front of you, arms fully extended.

Form:
Raise the bar up high, until it is even with your chin. Elbows will be higher than your hands. Hold, then slowly lower to the start position. Do not sway back and forth to raise the weight. This exercise may be done with dumbells as well.

Cheating:
To squeeze out extra repetitions at muscle failure, the leg may be used to help propel the bar from starting position.

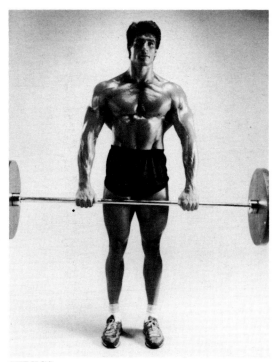
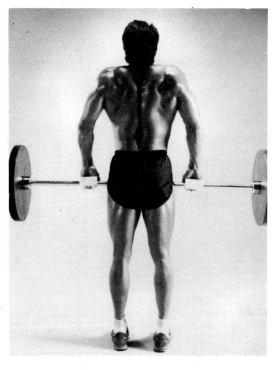

SHRUGS

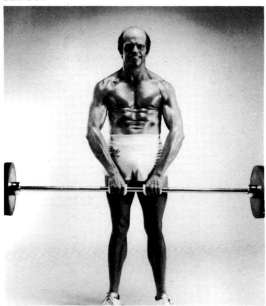
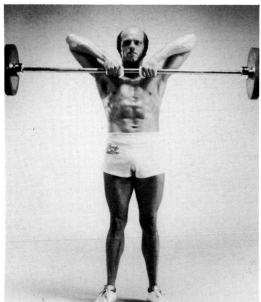

UPRIGHT ROWING

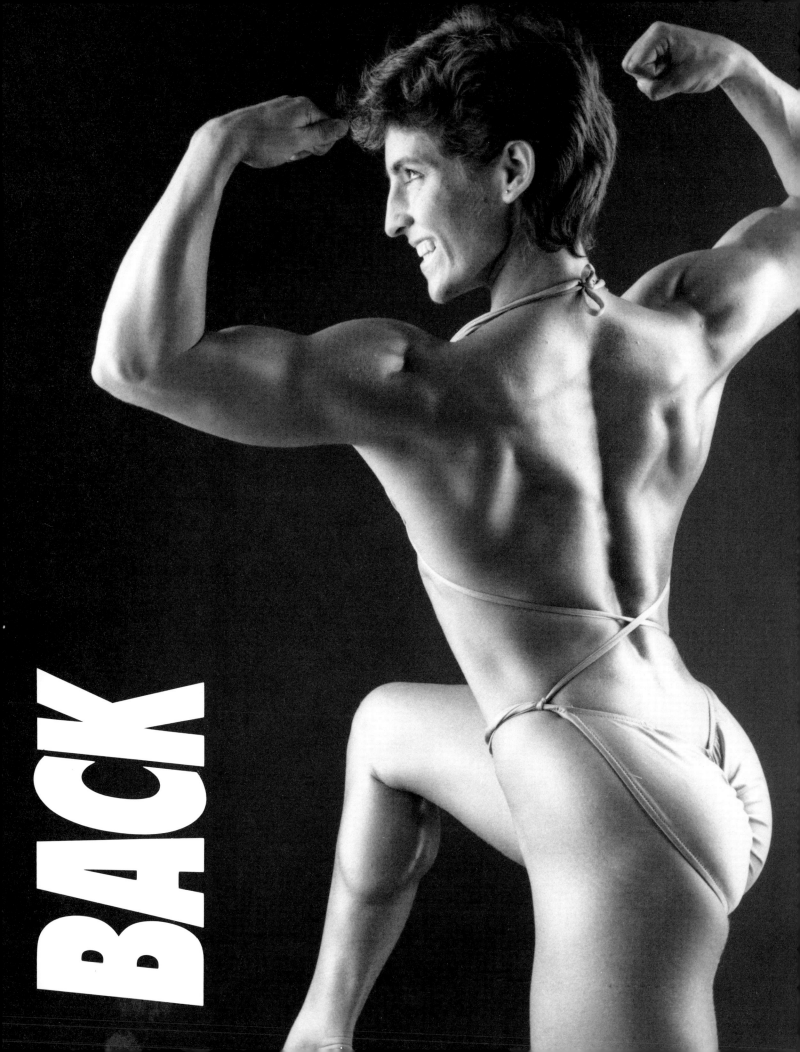

BACK

DEAD LIFT

Purpose:
To strengthen the lower back, aid in extension and moves of the trunk. The dead lift gives support for most other standing and sitting exercises.

Muscle Group:
Erector Spinae.

Secondary Support Groups:
Biceps femoris, trapezius.

Equipment:
Barbell, wood block
(6 x 12 x 24 inches)

Position:
Stand on the wood block, feet less than shoulder width apart, so that arms do not touch the legs during the movement. Feet are positioned just under the bar. Grasp the bar at shoulder width, palms facing toward you.

Form:
Bend your knees to let the thigh muscles help you with the first lift off the floor. Keeping your back straight and your head up, stand up straight, using the muscles of the lower back. Lower the bar to just touch the floor, then start it back up again. Keep the legs straight now and get maximum stretch and use of the biceps femoris while stressing the lower back.

Pointers:
1. An alternating grip of one palm facing in and one out helps to prevent the bar from rolling.
2. Flex at the top of the lift, pulling shoulders back as far as you can, chest out.
3. Standing on the block gives a fuller range of motion and a better stretch of the hamstrings.
4. In the beginning, you may not be able to stretch enough to let the barbell touch the floor. Go as far as you can.
5. A pair of lat straps or chiro grips may be used to assist the grips.

CAUTION!
A warm-up is mandatory. Do some bent-over toe touches and dead lift a very light weight to warm up the lower back. Do not attempt a dead lift at the beginning of the workout. Increase the weight gradually. Do not perform to muscle failure. This could cause low back injury. If you have a low back problem, consult your chiropractor and have it corrected before attempting heavy weights.

Variations:
1. Beginners may bend the legs slightly.
2. Standing on a bench will enable you to achieve a greater stretch than standing on the block.

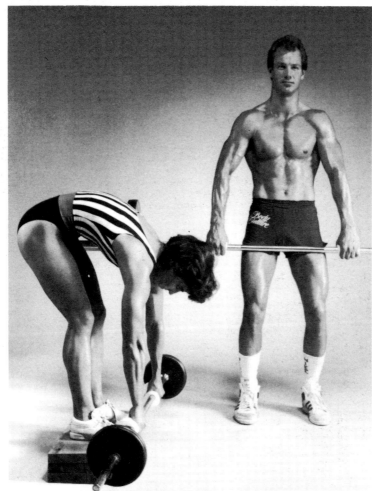

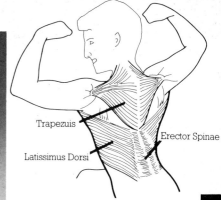

Trapezuis

Latissimus Dorsi

Erector Spinae

WEIGHTS

CHINS

Purpose:
To strengthen and develop the lower and upper back. This aids in all pulling actions.

Muscle Groups:
Latissimus dorsi, teres major, sternal portion of pectoralis major.

Secondary Support Groups:
Biceps and forearms.

Position:
The bar should be at a height just above your outstretched arm. Jump up and grab the bar with one of the grips described below. Bend the knees; this helps you to arch the back. The latissimus dorsi cannot be fully contracted unless the back is arched.

The grips: 1. Pronated (palms facing forward) and wider than shoulder width apart places the arm in a weaker position for chinning and stresses the latissimus dorsi.
2. Supinated (palms toward you) and shoulder width is a strong position for working on biceps.
3. Supinated with parallel grips (palms facing each other) not more than 25 inches apart enables you to work the latissimus dorsi harder.

Form:
Pull your body up until either your upper chest or trapezius touches the bar. Lower yourself to the hanging position slowly enough to be in control.

Variations:
1. Pull chest up to the bar with supinated grip. This stimulates the lower lats more.
2. Pull trapezius to the bar, using a pronated grip, to stimulate upper lats.
3. Generally, a wider grip works the upper lats, a narrow grip (on a V-bar) works the lower lats.

Pointers:
1. Remember to arch the back.
2. Use the hand grip which suits you best.
3. A training partner may hold a beginner's feet to help him.
4. Negative repetitions may be used by beginners who cannot pull themselves up, and by the more advanced to add stress at the end of a set. Stand on a bench to get the chin above the bar and do only the lowering phase of the exercise.
5. The wearing of a weighted belt increases resistance.
6. Do not swing the body or pump the legs.

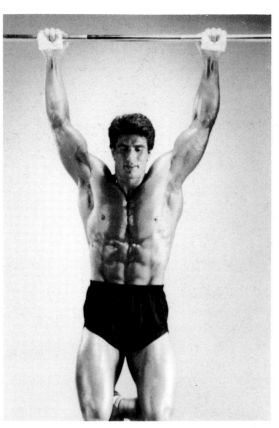

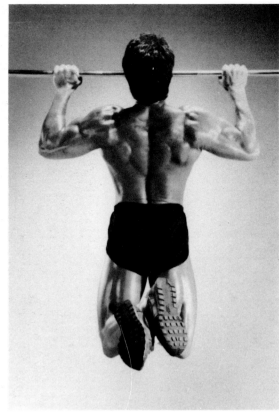

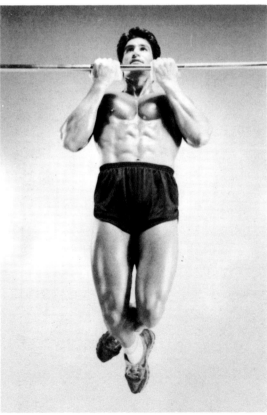

BENT-OVER ROWING

Muscle Group:
Latissimus dorsi, trapezius, erector spinae, biceps and brachialis.

Secondary Support Groups:
Posterior deltoid and forearms.

Equipment:
Barbell, wood block.

Position:
Feet wider apart than shoulder width. Bend over the bar and take a grip with palms facing toward you, about 24 inches apart. Bend the knees slightly, with the arms straight. Upper body is parallel to the floor. The back remains straight, except at the top of the exercise. If the barbell is still touching the floor in this position, stand on a wood block.

Form:
Pull the barbell in toward your chest, moving the upper arm parallel to the body. Hold this top position, arch the back a little and flex your lats even more if you can.

Variations:
1. A wide grip of more than 24 inches emphasizes the upper lats, a medium grip the middle lats and a 14-inch narrow grip the lower lats.
2. The head may be extended forward, or you may look down. See which position best effects the area on which you are working.
3. The higher the position of the bar on the chest at the top of the exercise, the higher the lats are worked.

HYPEREXTENSIONS

Muscle Group:
Erector spinae.

Secondary Support Group:
Hamstrings.

Equipment:
Bench, wood block.

Position:
Lie prone on a bench, raised at one end with a large wood block (6 x 12 x 24 inches), with your upper torso hanging over the raised end. Hook your feet under the bench, or have a training partner hold them. Hands rest on your temples, elbows flared out.

Form:
Flex forward from the waist as far down as the height of the bench permits. Contract the muscles of the lower back to extend the torso upward. Arch the back as far as possible abover the horizontal, for complete contraction. Do 20 to 25 repetitions.

Variation:
You may twist and arch to one side, then the other, to stress the erector spinae at a different angle.

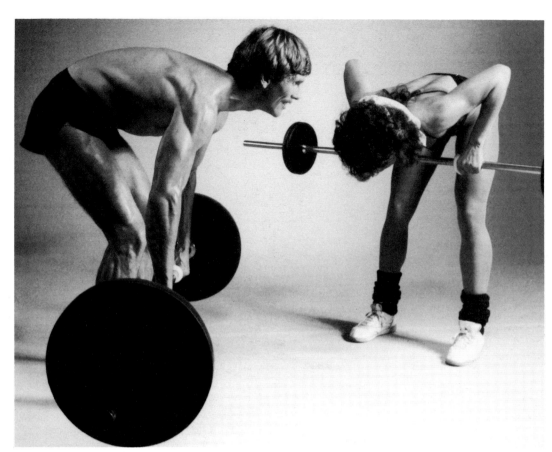

BENT-OVER ROWING

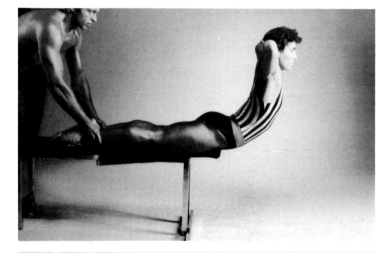

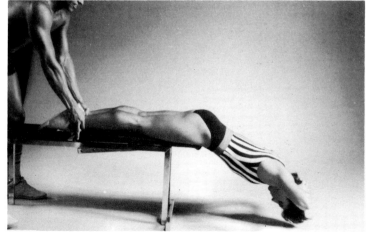

HYPEREXTENSIONS

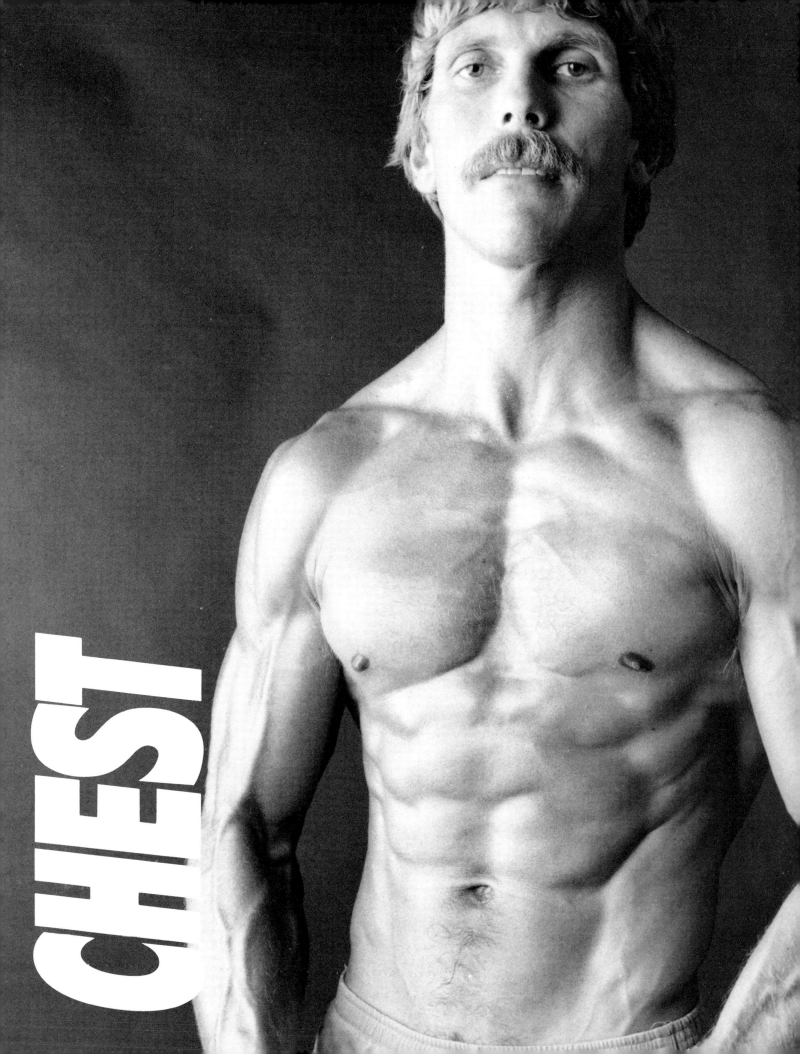

CHEST

BENCH PRESS

Purpose:
To develop the chest and upper body. This aids in all pushing movements.

Muscle Groups:
Upper and lower pectoralis, anterior deltoid.

Secondary Support Groups:
Triceps, latissimus dorsi.

Equipment:
Bench with supporting rack, barbell or two dumbells and training partner.

NOTE: A warm-up is important before this exercise.
We recommend the door stretch, elbows back and full range bench press with light weight.

Grips:
Try for a comfortable grip, with palms facing the feet. Exact spacing depends upon the individual. Generally, a narrow grip, less than shoulder width, with the bar meeting the chest below the nipple emphasizes the inner and lower pectorals and the triceps. A grip of shoulder width and wider, with the bar high on the chest emphasizes the upper and outer pectorals and anterior deltoids.

Position:
With the bar loaded to desired weight and placed in the rack, lie supine on the bench with your chin directly under the bar, feet flat on the floor. Grasp the bar at the desired width. As the weight used increases, the training partner will need to assist you in getting the weight into starting position.
The spotter's position is at the head of the bench, to safely assist in the placement of the weight at the start and end of a set.

Form:
After the weight is taken off the rack, the bar should be directly above the shoulder and upper chest, arms straight, perpendicular to the floor. Lower the bar to the chest and, with a continuous motion, pull it back up to the starting position with the pectoral muscles – not by pushing with the arms. The elbow will go out to the side as the weight descends. Keep your upper arm at 90 degrees to your torso. Keep your head and buttocks on the bench. Do not push with the feet. Use only the upper body muscles and do not arch your back.

CAUTION!
Do not hold your breath during the press, as it is possible to black out and drop the bar on your chest or neck.

Pointers:
1. If you find you are pushing with the feet and legs, try a new weight, or take your feet off the floor, with the legs raised at 90 degrees and knees bent. This will also keep the back flat and the buttocks down.
2. For maximum benefit, don't lock the arms at the top of the move, flex the pectorals, instead.
3. If the elbows are creeping forward in the down position, the emphasis switches to the anterior deltoid.
4. Visualize the pectoral muscles squeezing toward the center, pulling the arms up.

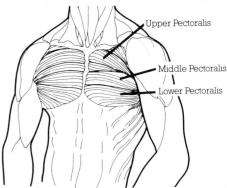

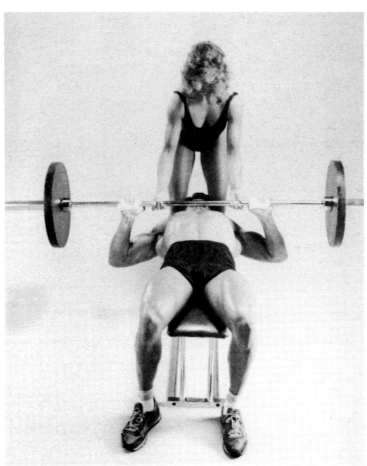

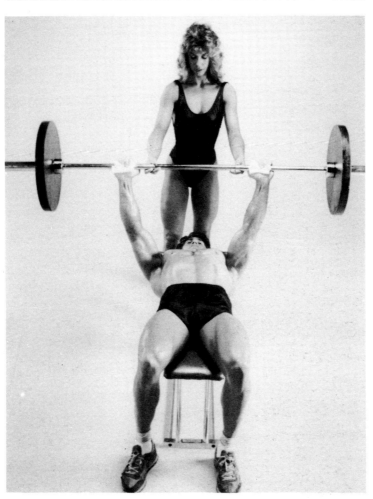

INCLINE BENCH PRESS

Muscle Group:
Upper pectorals.

Secondary Support Groups:
Anterior deltoids and triceps.

Equipment:
Incline bench, set at 45 degrees and barbell or dumbells.

Position:
Sit on an incline bench with your feet on the floor. The barbell grip variations are the same as for the bench press and the bar is across the upper chest.
If you are using dumbells, raise them to slightly more than shoulder width, with the palms facing out, away from you.

Form:
Pull the weight straight up to arm's length, so that the inside of the dumbells touch or until the bar is perpendicular to the shoulders. This is done by contracting the upper pectorals from the outside-in, toward the sternum. Concentrate on flexing the upper pectorals for one second, then lower the weight to starting position.

Pointer:
Doing the exercise with dumbells gives a fuller stretch of the pectorals muscles, as the arms can pull back lower than with the barbell. Remember to keep the elbows as far back as possible. If you feel it in your shoulders, your elbows are too far forward.

DECLINE PRESS

Muscle Group:
Lower pectoralis.

Secondary Support Group:
Anterior and middle deltoids, triceps and latissimus dorsi.

Equipment:
Bench, wood block (6 x 12 x 24 inches), barbell or dumbells.

Position:
With one end of the bench on the block, lie supine on the bench with your head at the lower end. Hook the knees over the other end. If you have an adjustable bench, set it at 30 degrees.
1. If using a barbell, have a training partner hand you the weight. Take a palms-forward grip and hold the bar at arm's length. A wide grip will work the outer pectorals, a narrow grip the inner pectorals. A spotter is advisable when using the barbell.
2. If using dumbells, get the weights to your shoulders, palms facing forward, as above.

Form:
1. Lower the barbell to the lower chest, below the nipples, keeping elbows out at 90 degrees to the body. The head stays down, the buttocks on the bench. Do not arch the back. Then squeeze the pectorals from the outside to the center, contracting the muscles totally to raise the weight to starting position. At the top of the move, squeeze the lower pectorals for one second.
2. Pull the dumbells perpendicular to a fully extended arm's length and have the weights almost touch at the top. Flex the lower pectorals at the top for one second, then lower again.

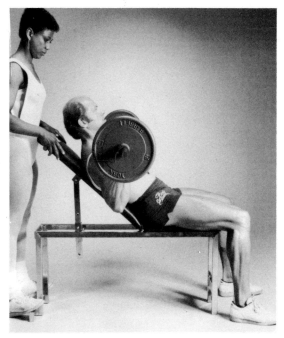 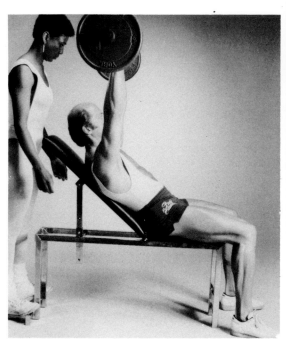

INCLINE BENCH PRESS

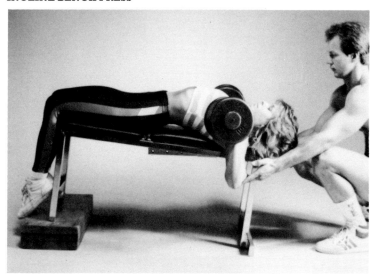

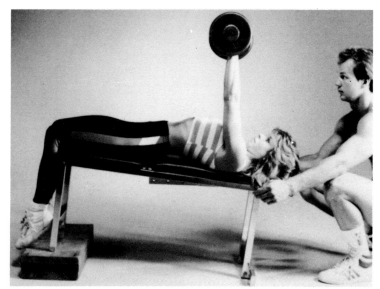

DECLINE PRESS

DUMBELL FLIES

Muscle Group:
Outer pectoralis.

Equipment:
Flat bench, dumbell.

Position:
Lie supine on a bench, with dumbells in your hands. Raise the dumbells above your chest, arching the arms and allowing the weights to touch. Palms face each other.

Form:
Keeping the arms bowed, as though you were hugging a barrel, lower the weights as far as possible to the side to stretch the pectoral muscles. Raise the dumbells back to the starting position using only the pectorals and squeeze for one second.

Pointers:
Keeping the elbows bent eliminates overstressing of the elbow joints. Arch the chest upward in the full stretch position, but keep your head on the bench.

Variations:
1. Incline flies will stress the upper and outer pectorals.
2. Decline flies will stress the lower and outer pectorals.

PULL OVER

Muscle Groups:
Pectorals, latissimus dorsi, serratus.

Equipment:
Flat bench and dumbell.

Position:
Lie across a bench with only your shoulders and upper back supported, and your knees bent and feet flat on the floor. Your body is parallel to the floor. Have a training partner pass you the dumbell. With palms facing up, grasp the inside of one weight at one end of the dumbell. Raise it to a vertical position above your chest.

Form:
Lower the weight with a straight arm, at the same time arching your back and dropping your hips. Lower the weight as far as possible to maximize the stretch. With a conscious flexing of the pectorals, latissimus dorsi and serratus, pull the dumbell up and raise the hips up simultaneously. This is also an excellent stretch for the rib cage.

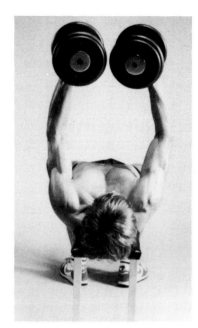
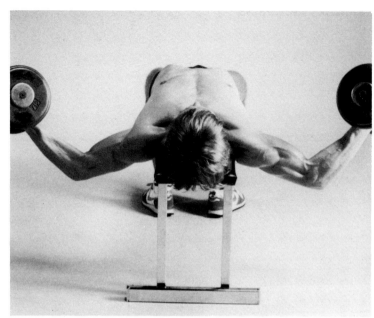

DUMBELL FLIES

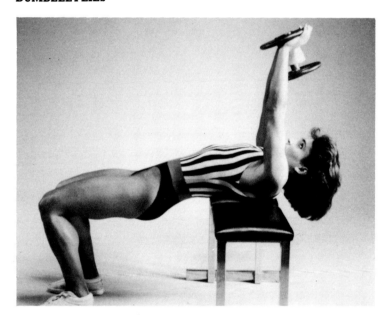
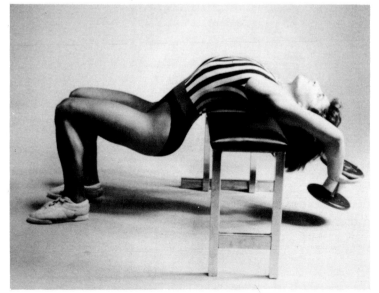

PULL OVER

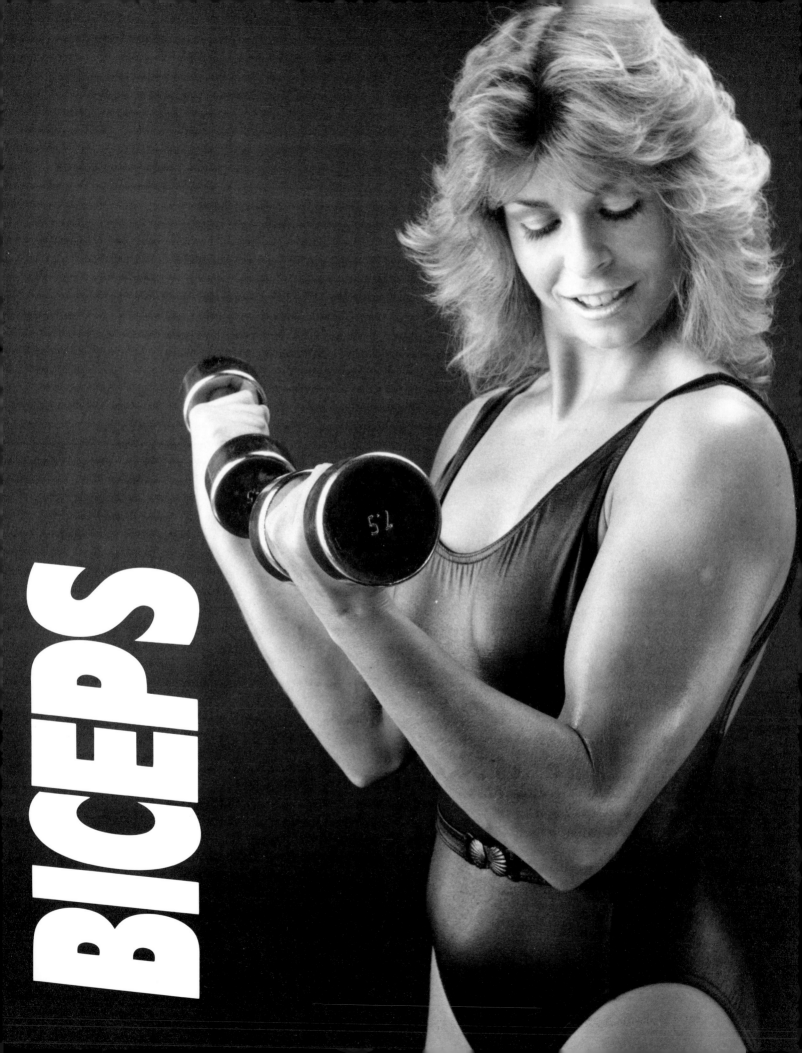

BICEPS

BARBELL CURL

Purpose:
To improve strength in movements of flexing the elbow and supination of the forearm – turning the hand from a palm-down to palm-up position.

Muscle Groups:
Biceps, brachialis, brachiordialis.

Secondary Support Groups:
Forearm (radial and ulnar flexors), a combination of wrist, finger and elbow flexors.

Equipment:
Barbell. Weightlifting belt optional.

Position:
All grips used have the palms up. A narrow grip, hands six to eight inches apart, works the outer bicep. A medium grip of 12 to 14 inches works the middle bicep. A wide grip of 24 to 26 inches works the inner bicep. You stand erect, feet shoulder width apart, with the bar resting on your thighs and hands set in your chosen grip. A spotter may be facing you during the exercise.

Form:
Move elbows slightly to the front of the body. Slowly raise the bar in a circular motion toward the chest. When the bar has reached the upper position, raise the elbows as far as possible to squeeze a total contraction at the top. Lower the bar to starting position under total control. Use different grips for variation.

Pointers:
Don't swing the upper body or the weight to get momentum. Keep the elbows in until the finish of the curl, then raise. Make use of the negative phase of the movement, as this is very beneficial to development. When the muscle is exhausted, have the training partner help move the weight to the top position and concentrate on two or three more negative repetitions. Visualize the bicep working and growing stronger.

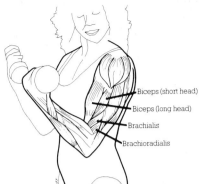

Biceps (short head)
Biceps (long head)
Brachialis
Brachioradialis

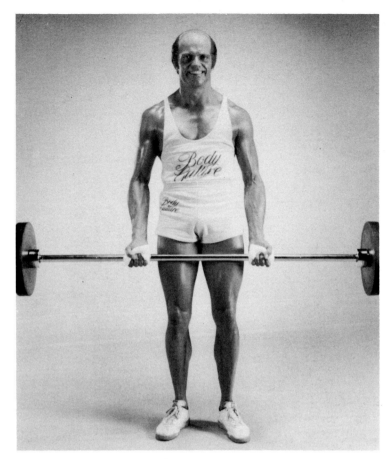

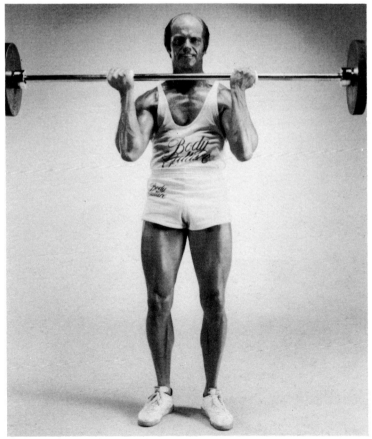

ALTERNATING CURLS

Muscle Groups:
Biceps, brachialis, forearm flexors.

Equipment:
Dumbells.

Position:
Same as for standing curl.

Form:
Start to curl your right dumbell upward, while rotating the wrist, to finish with the palm facing upward (supination). Raise the elbow and flex, as in standing curl. As you lower the right dumbell, raise the left and repeat the motions. This may be done in a sitting position. This exercise allows you to concentrate on one arm at a time.

CONCENTRATION CURL

Muscle Group:
Biceps, particularly the bicep peak.

Equipment:
Dumbell, bench.

Position:
Sit on the end of a bench, feet wide apart, and bend forward. Lean slightly to the right. Support the left hand on the left knee, but let the right arm suspend.

Form:
With dumbell in the right hand, slowly curl the extended arm upwards. Supinate slightly to finish with the palm up. Do not move the elbow position at the top of the curl. Squeeze out a full contraction for one or two seconds, then lower the dumbell. Do the required number of repetitions, then switch to the other arm.

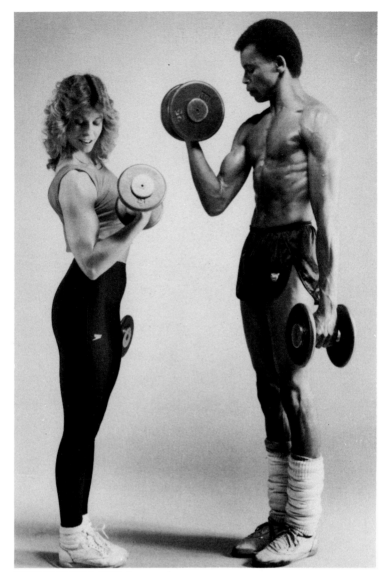

ALTERNATING CURLS

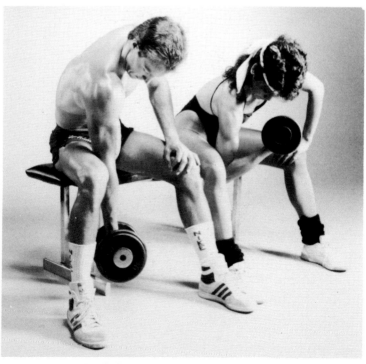

CONCENTRATION CURL

INCLINE CURL

Muscle Groups:
Biceps, brachialis, forearm flexors.

Equipment:
Dumbells, incline bench.

Position:
Set the bench at a 30° - 45° incline.
Sit on it with a dumbell in each hand,
hanging straight down to each side.

Form:
The same as Alternating Curls, or you
may do both arms at the same time.

Variation:
Flare your hands out to the side to hit
different angles of the bicep.

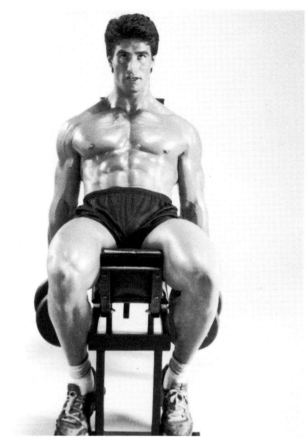

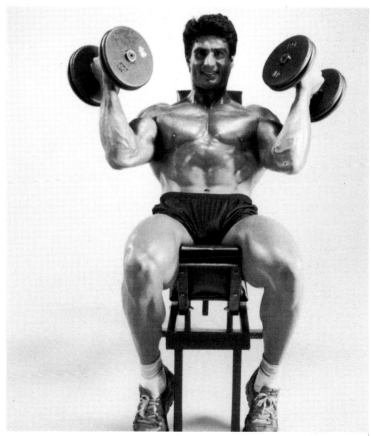

61

TRICEPS

TRICEP EXTENSIONS
(Supine, Standing and Sitting French Press)

Purpose:
To improve the power in extension of the elbow joint. These movements are used in throwing sports such as baseball and football.

Muscle Group:
Inner head of triceps.

Secondary Support Group:
Long head and lateral head of triceps.

Equipment:
Bench and barbell.

Position:
1. Supine – lie on the bench with arms straight up.
2. Standing – push bar overhead to straight-arm position.
3. Sitting – push bar up to a straight-arm position.
The grip for all three tricep extensions is with palms up and thumbs back, hands six to 10 inches apart.
A spotter should stand facing the lifter, to assist in the last few repetitions or in negative repetitions.

Form:
1. Supine – lower the barbell in a semi-circular motion, keeping the upper arm vertical until the bar almost touches the forehead. Press the bar back up to starting position.
2. Standing and Sitting – push the bar up to straight-arm position and lower it to behind the neck. Keep the elbows as high as possible. Squeeze the tricep at the top position.

Pointers:
1. Warm up by extending the arms and flexing the triceps or by doing a few repetitions with light weights. Warm-up is not necessary if this exercise follows presses for shoulders and chest.
2. Don't rest when the arm is fully extended, but squeeze the triceps for a maximum contraction. Keep the upper arm still and keep the elbows tucked in as close as possible.

Variations:
Reverse the grip to do what is known as a tricep curl. This places more stress on the long head of the triceps. Hand position is about shoulder width.

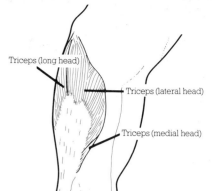

Triceps (long head)
Triceps (lateral head)
Triceps (medial head)

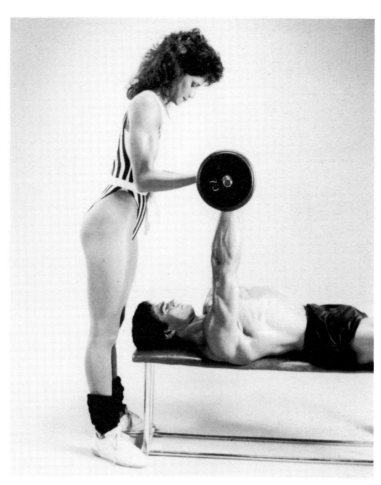

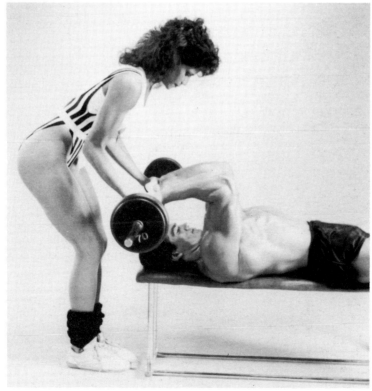

ONE ARM EXTENSIONS

Muscle Group:
Triceps.

Equipment:
Bench and dumbell.

Position:
Sit on the edge of the bench with a dumbell in one hand. Raise it over the head with the arm fully extended and the palm facing inward.

Form:
Lower the dumbell behind your head until the palm is at the base of the neck. Keep the upper arm against the side of your head, and motionless throughout the exercise. Extend the arm back to upright position and flex the tricep at the top. Do a full set and switch hands.

Variations:
1. Standing position.
2. Sitting with back supported.
3. Using one heavy dumbell and two hands.
4. Exercising both arms at the same time.

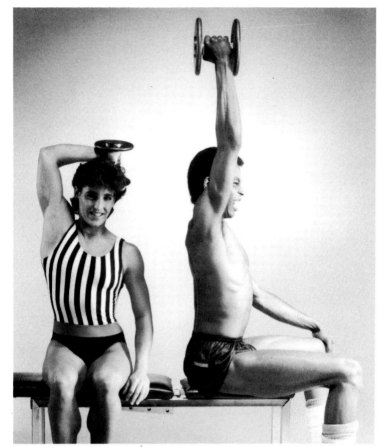

ONE ARM EXTENSIONS

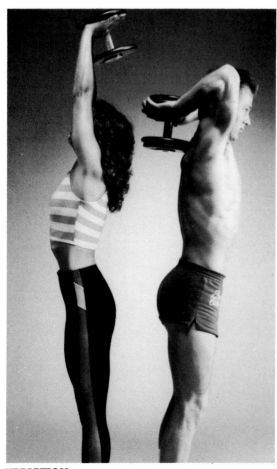

VARIATION

BENCH DIP

Muscle Group:
Triceps.

Equipment:
Two benches or one bench and something slightly higher on which the feet will rest.

Position:
Place the benches far enough apart to permit you to rest your feet on one and hands on the other, with enough space to lower your body between them. The feet are together on one bench and your hands are behind your back. Grasp the edge of the bench and extend your arms. The closer the hands are together, the more difficult the exercise.

Form:
Bend your arm and lower your body as far down as possible. Upper arms should be parallel to the floor. Push yourself back up to arms-extended position again and flex triceps. Lower again. For added resistance, place a barbell plate or dumbell in you lap.

Variations:
Place two or three weight plates in your lap and have a training partner remove them one at a time when you cannot raise the weight. Keep going until all have been removed and you cannot rise again. Do this for your last set to "burn" the triceps.

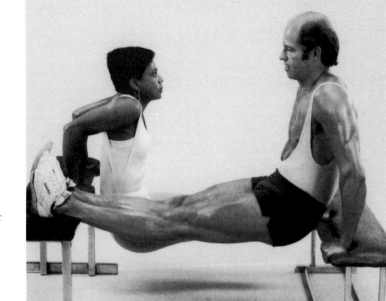

BENCH DIP

KICK BACKS

Muscle Group:
Outer head of tricep.

Equipment:
Dumbells.

Position:
Grasp a dumbell in the right hand. Bend over a flat bench, so the torso is parallel to the floor and support yourself on the bench with the left hand. Raise your right upper arm to a position parallel to your upper body and keep it there for the entire exercise. The forearm hangs down, vertically.

Form:
Extend the forearm back until it, too, reaches a parallel position, in a straight line with the upper arm. Squeeze the tricep and hold for one second, then slowly lower the forearm to start position. Do a full set, then switch to the other arm.

Variation:
You may exercise both arms at the same time, placing the head against a support to keep the body from swinging.

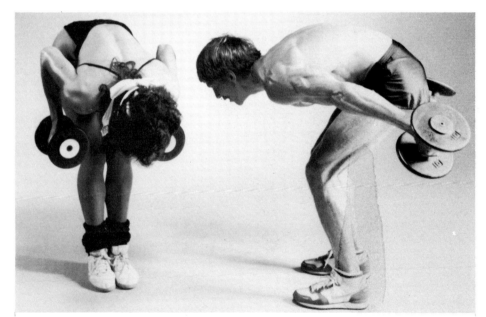

KICK BACKS

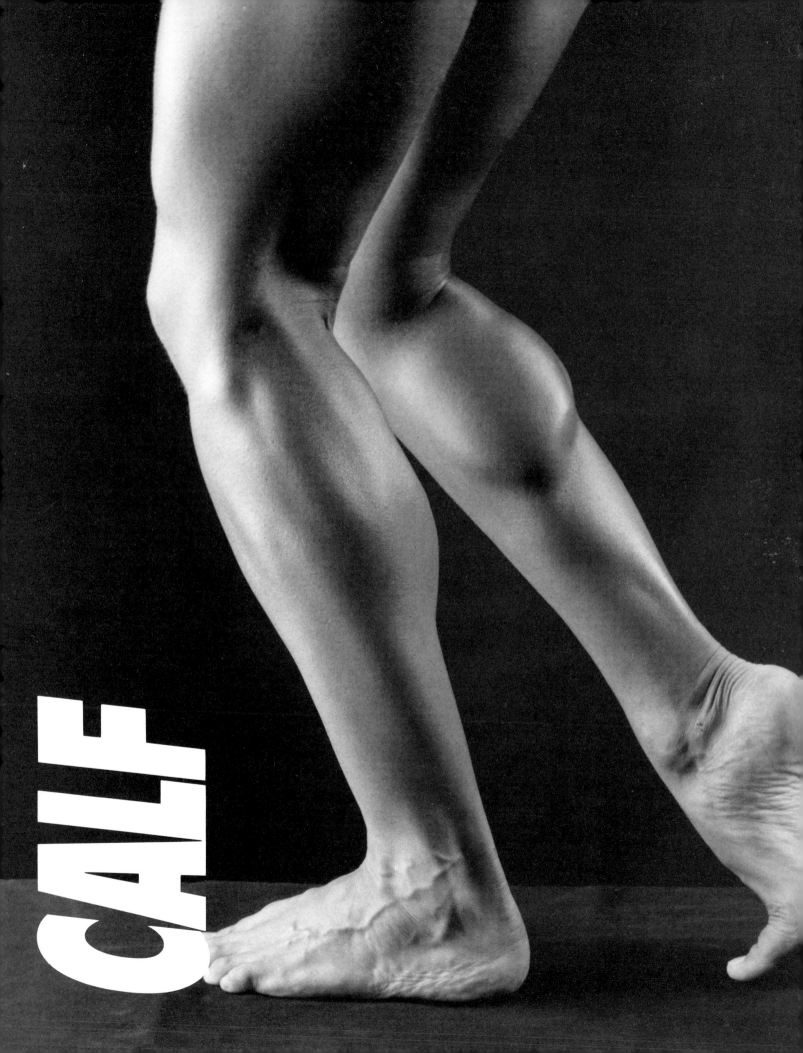

CALF

CALF RAISE BARBELL

Purpose:
To improve ankle joint extension. This provides propulsion in walking, running and jumping.

Muscle Groups:
Gastrocnemius (calf).

Equipment:
Barbell and wood block (one edge sanded down for better grip and fuller stretch).

Position:
Warm up for the exercise by stretching the calf muscles while on the wood block, doing some calf raises with little or no weight, or by skipping. Place the bar across the shoulders and back as in the squat lifts. Stand on one edge of the block with the balls of the feet on the wood and the heels off. Feet point forward, shoulder width apart. A spotter may help with balance.

Form:
Lower your heels as far as possible, then rise up, using the calf and soleus muscles to full extension. Flex them at the top of the move. Repeat 15 to 20 times.

Variations:
Foot positions – toes turned out affects the inner calf muscle; toes turned in affects the outer calf muscle.
You may also exercise one calf at a time, using a dumbell in one hand and supporting yourself with the other hand.

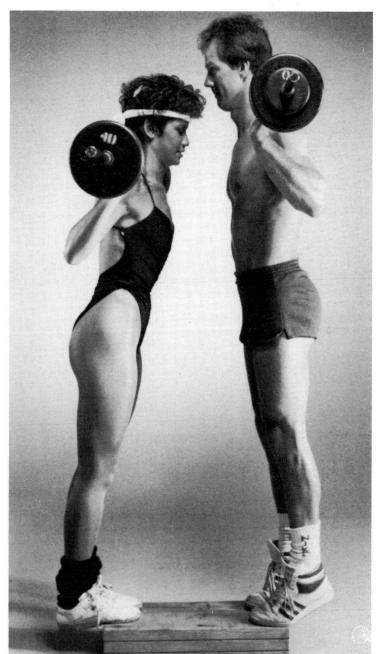

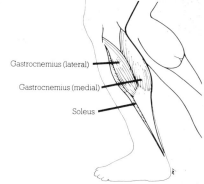

Gastrocnemius (lateral)

Gastrocnemius (medial)

Soleus

DONKEY CALF RAISE

Muscle Groups:
Gastrocnemius (calf).

Equipment:
Calf block (6 x 12 x 24 inches) and training partner.

Position:
Stand with the balls of your feet on the calf block and bend forward with the upper body almost parallel to the floor. Use the hand to support yourself on a bench or something similar. The training partner sits on your hips, legs astride you.

Form:
Lower your heels to a full stretch of the calf, then raise up to full extension (full contraction). Do 15 to 20 repetitions.

Variations:
Use different toe positions to work different parts of the calf, as noted in calf raises, above.

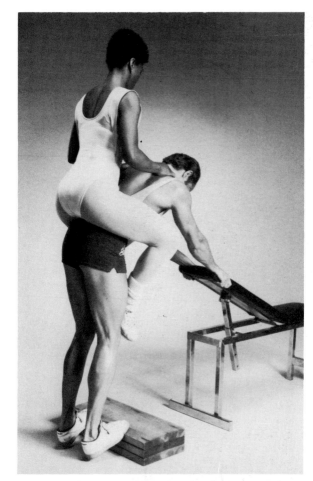

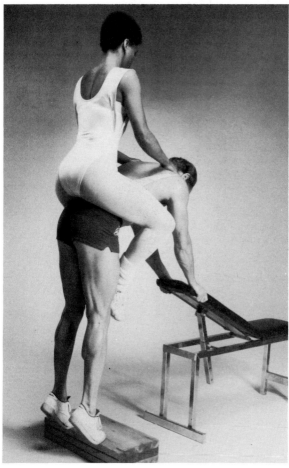

SITTING SOLEUS RAISE

Muscle Group:
Soleus. This muscle, located under the calf, can only be fully contracted when the leg is bent at 90 degrees.

Equipment:
Barbell or dumbell, bench, wood block.

Position:
Sit on the edge of the bench and hold the barbell across the lower thigh, three inches above the knee. Place a set of chiro chips between the bar and your thigh for comfort. Rest your toes and the balls of your feet on the edge of the block, leaving the heels unsupported.

Form:
Raise the heels as high as possible, slowly, by contracting the soleus. At the top, fully contract the soleus and calf muscles. Hold and slowly lower to a full stretch of the calf and soleus. Do 15 to 20 repetitions per set. Do not lean back and pull up the weights with your hands.

Variations:
A single-leg soleus raise is possible when a dumbell is used on one knee. Vary the toe positions to change the emphasis from inner soleus (toes in) to outer soleus (toes out).

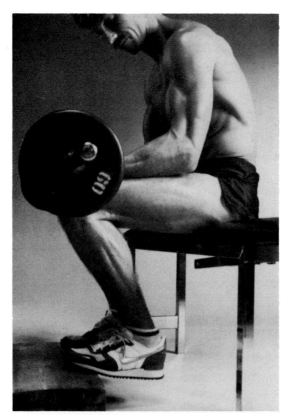

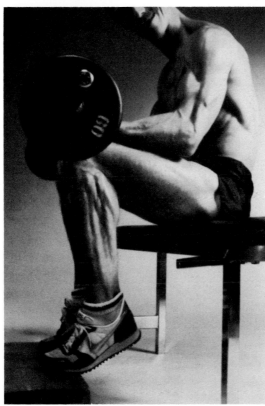

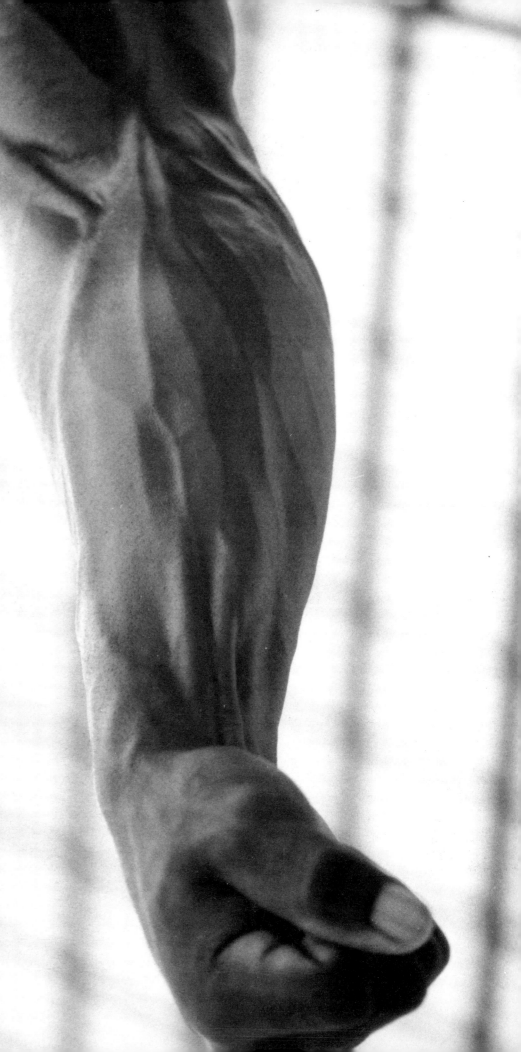

FOREARM

WRIST CURL

Purpose:
To improve flexion and extension of the wrist. This is used in gripping objects and in pronation and supination of the hand.

Muscle Groups:
Inside forearm group (flexors); outside forearm group (extensors).

Equipment:
Bench and dumbells.

Positions:
1. Hands with palms up, 12 inches apart and thumb under the bar. The prime movers will be the flexors.
2. Hands with palms down, same spacing. The prime mover will be the extensors.
Sit on the edge of the bench, resting forearms on the thighs and use either grip to hold the bar. The wrists are extended out, over the knees.

Form:
1. If palms are up, lower the weight by extending the wrists downward and rolling the bar down to the fingers by opening the grip. Close the grip and fully flex the wrist.
2. If palms are down, lower the weight by flexing the wrist. Open the grip a little for full flexion, then close the grip and fully extend the wrist. Alternate grips.
You may use a dumbell to do one arm at a time.

Pointers:
1. Don't lift the forearms off your thighs.
2. Don't assist with a push from the calves.
3. Weight is usually less with palms down than palms up.
4. With palms up, keep the thumb under the bar for more contraction of the flexors.

REVERSE CURL

Muscle Groups:
Forearm extensors, biceps and brachialis.

Equipment:
Barbell

Position:
Stand comfortably, with palms-down grip on the barbell (overgrip) and the hands a bit less than shoulder width apart. The arms are extended down in front of the body.

Form:
Slowly raise the bar up by bending the elbows. Keep the upper arm down and close to the body. Arch the bar up by using the forearm and upper arms to raise the bar to a fully flexed position. Lower slowly to start position.
Keep the body erect. Do not swing the weight with your upper body. Narrowing the grip changes the emphasis slightly.

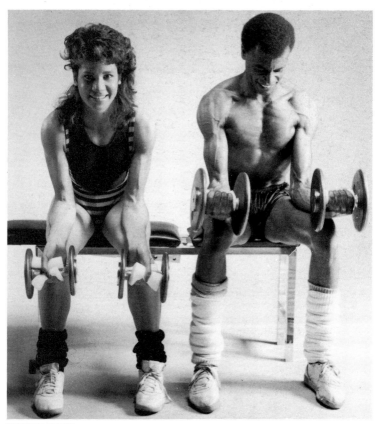

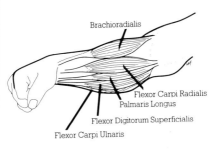

Brachioradialis
Flexor Carpi Radialis
Palmaris Longus
Flexor Digitorum Superficialis
Flexor Carpi Ulnaris

WRIST CURL

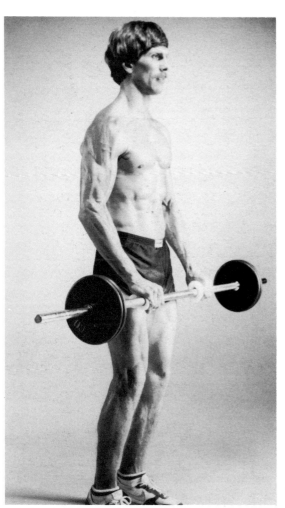

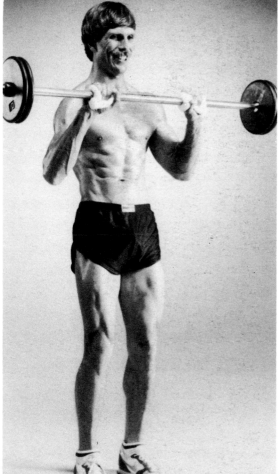

REVERSE CURL

BEHIND THE BACK
WRIST CURL

Muscle Group:
Forearm flexors.

Equipment:
Barbell, bench press rack.

Position:
Place a moderately weighted barbell in the rack at waist height. Back up to the weight and grasp the bar behind you, with hands shoulder width apart. Thumbs and palms are under the bar. Raise the bar off the rack and move forward slightly.

Form:
Keep your arms straight down and flex your wrists up and back as far as possible. Lower slowly, until the bar is supported only by the fingers, then curl the fingers and wrist back up again.

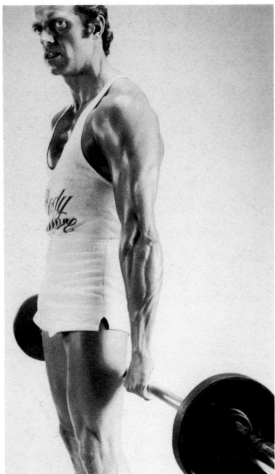

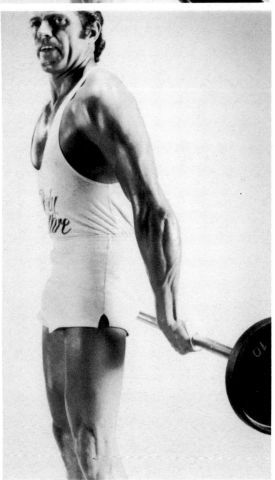

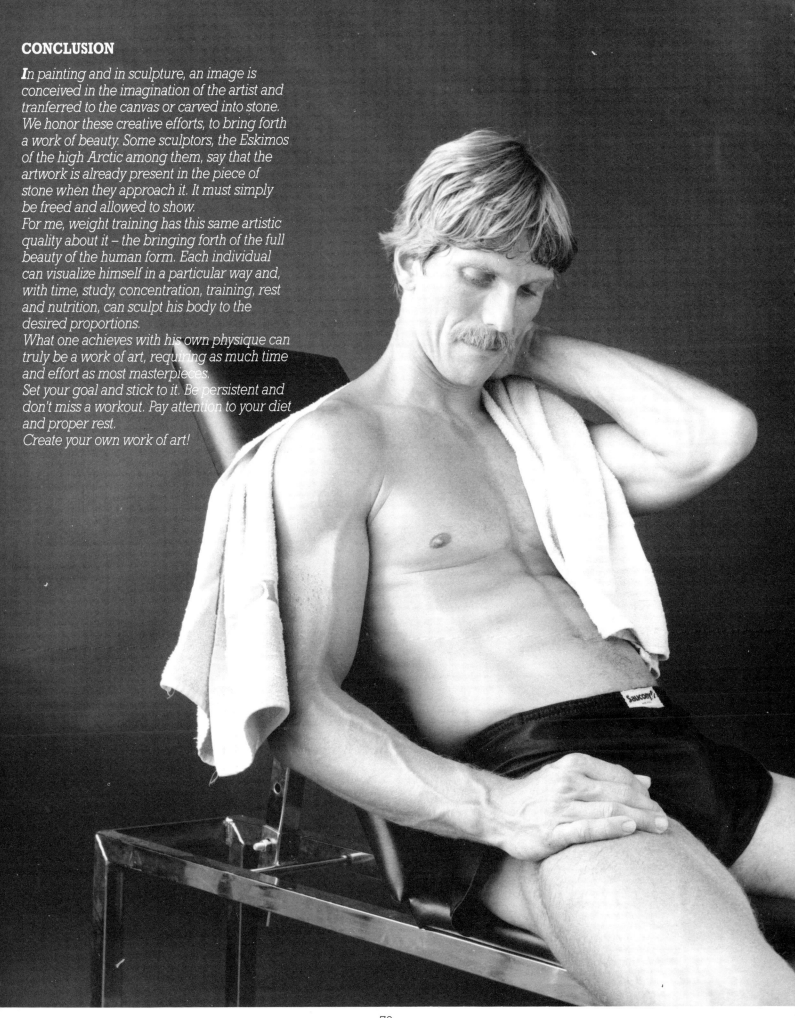

CONCLUSION

In painting and in sculpture, an image is
conceived in the imagination of the artist and
tranferred to the canvas or carved into stone.
We honor these creative efforts, to bring forth
a work of beauty. Some sculptors, the Eskimos
of the high Arctic among them, say that the
artwork is already present in the piece of
stone when they approach it. It must simply
be freed and allowed to show.
For me, weight training has this same artistic
quality about it – the bringing forth of the full
beauty of the human form. Each individual
can visualize himself in a particular way and,
with time, study, concentration, training, rest
and nutrition, can sculpt his body to the
desired proportions.
What one achieves with his own physique can
truly be a work of art, requiring as much time
and effort as most masterpieces.
Set your goal and stick to it. Be persistent and
don't miss a workout. Pay attention to your diet
and proper rest.
Create your own work of art!

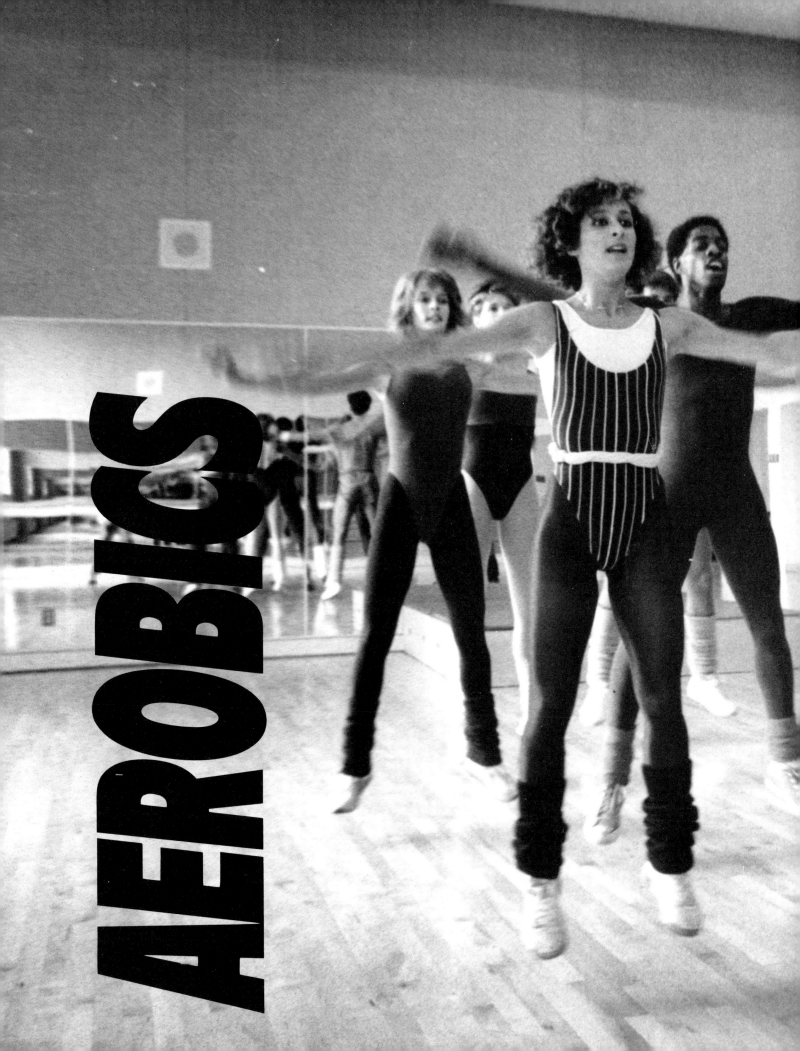

AEROBICS

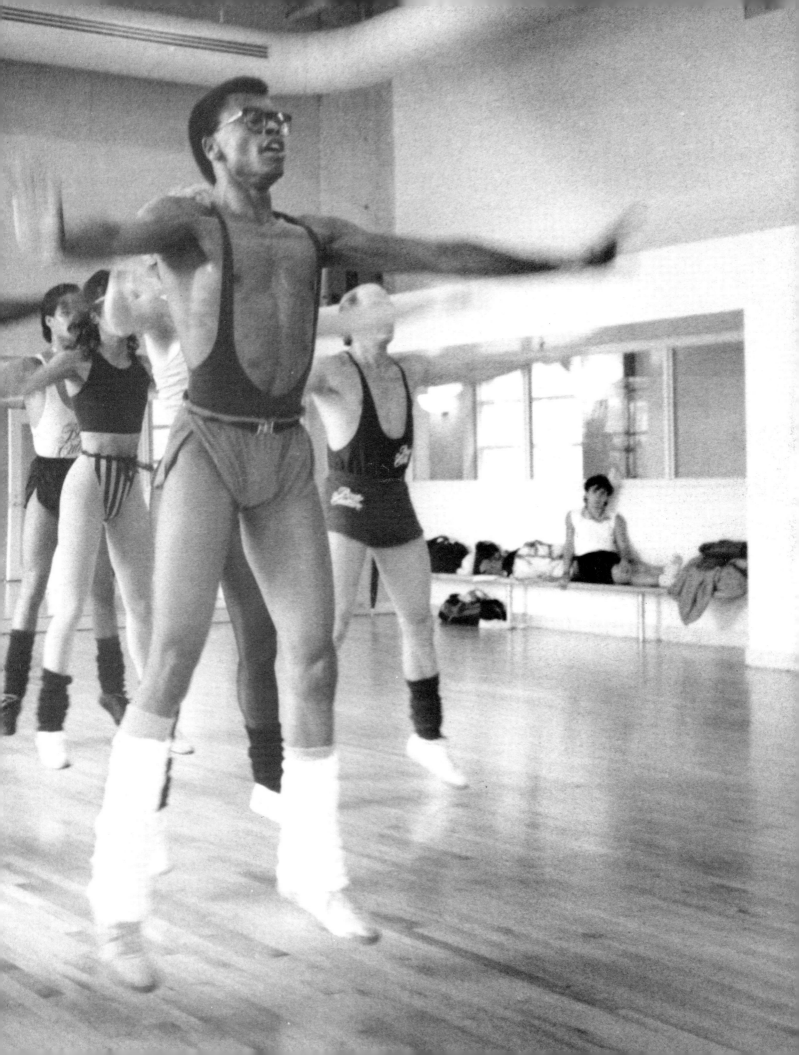

PURPOSE

A body that uses oxygen efficiently is a body that will function better and have more energy. Here is a brief list of the benefits of aerobic exercise.

- [ ] *it improves the anaerobic metabolism*
- [ ] *it improves the circulation (nutrients in, waste out)*
- [ ] *it improves oxygen transport through the body*
- [ ] *it increases your level of endurance*
- [ ] *it strengthens the heart as a muscle*
- [ ] *it expands the lung capacity*
- [ ] *it tones and develops muscles*
- [ ] *it burns off calories, rather than allowing them to accumulate as fat deposits*
- [ ] *it can offer stress relief from high pressure job situations or daily living.*

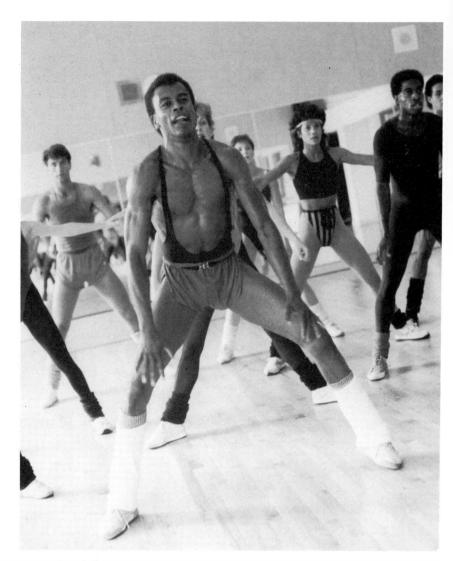

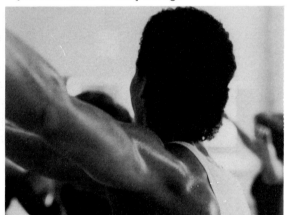

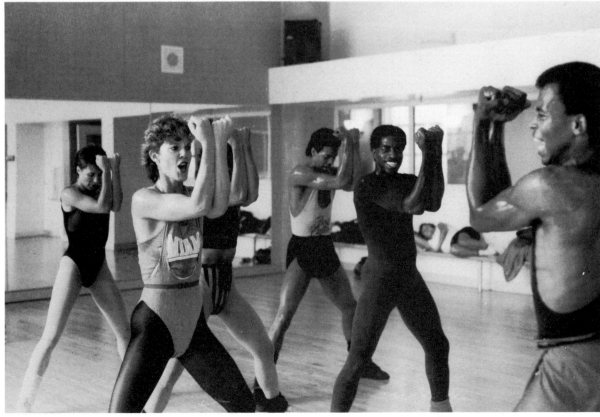

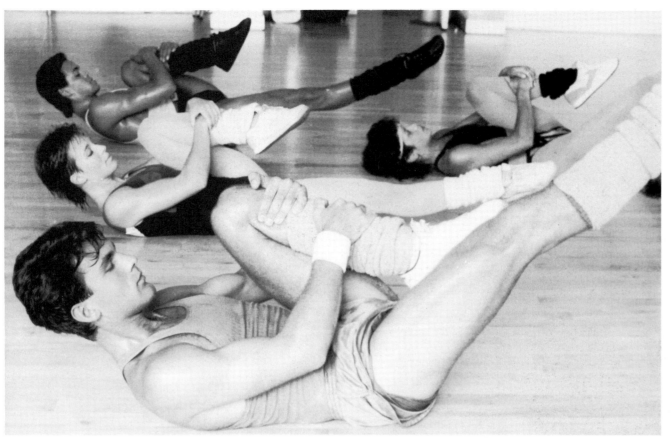

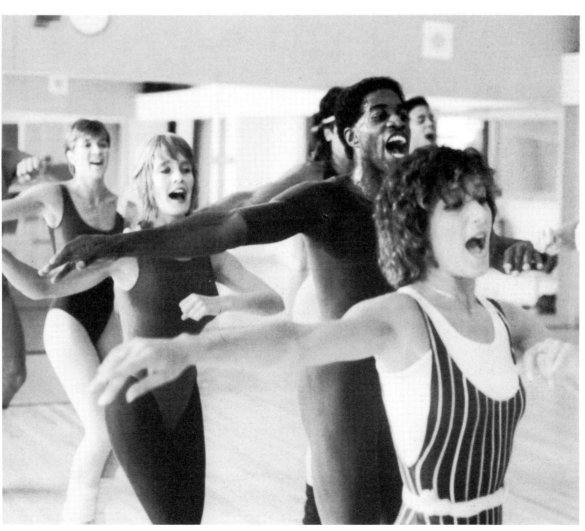

77

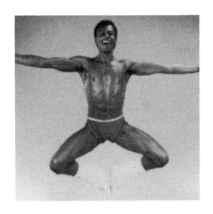

ALIGNMENT AND FOOT POSITIONS FOR WARM-UP

Points of technique for foot positions.

FIRST POSITION
Stand erect and tall, with feet together. Feel that you are trying to create space between each vertebra in the spinal column. The weight is forward on the toes. The top of the pelvis is tipped back to provide a lengthened lower back. This prevents hyperextension of the lower spine.

SECOND POSITION
Stand erect with the feet apart, approximately three to six inches wider than shoulder width. Again, the pelvis is tipped back to prevent hyperextension of the lower spine. Maintain the same tall feeling.

FOURTH POSITION
Stand erect and tall with the feet shoulder width apart. Place one foot in front of the body, as if to take a step forward. Right foot foward is called "fourth position, right side," and left foot forward is called "fourth position, left side."

PLIE -- *This term is borrowed from the French ballet repertoire and it means, simply, the bending of the legs. This basic exercise develops the muscles of the thighs, calves, ankles and feet. The action of the plie is slow and controlled. It serves to increase flexibility and strength in the tendons of the legs.*

As *the legs bend, the line of the thigh remains in line with the foot. The buttocks never drop below the level of the knees.*

When *doing a plie in the second position, the thighs open as the legs bend, so that a good stretch is achieved in the groin.*

Body alignment as checked from the front:
1. *The toe line is parallel to the front surface of the room.*
2. *The pelvic line is parallel to the front surface of the room.*
3. *The shoulder line is parallel to the front surface of the room.*
4. *The belt line is parallel to the floor.*
5. *Angles between toe, pelvic line and shoulder line must be kept as close as possible to zero, so as not to create torsion in the lower back.*
6. *The abdominal muscles, quadriceps and gluteus are used to maintain pelvic position.*
7. *When bending, the head stays in line laterally and frontally with the torso.*

Frontal *alignment is most important when doing exercises for the waist. The focus of the side stretches is up and out (45 degrees high), using fingertips to direct and focus the stretch. The idea is to limit the amount of lateral flexion in the spine, to prevent injury.*

BE CAREFUL NOT TO:
☐ *allow creation of angles between toe, pelvic and shoulder lines.*
☐ *allow for creation of angles between the front surface of the room and the toe, pelvic and shoulder lines. Stay square to the front.*
☐ *create an angle between the floor and the belt line. This indicates lateral pelvic tilt.*
☐ *cause lateral hyperflexion of the spine. If a person is in this position, he is probably using body weight to do the work and not stabilizing the pelvis with the abdominal muscles, quadriceps and gluteus.*

Body alignment, as checked from the side:
1. *The body is in a straight line, head to foot.*
2. *The weight is forward on the toes.*
3. *The pelvis is rotated back to lengthen the lower spine.*
4. *The belt line is parallel to the floor.*
5. *The chin line is elevated a few degrees above parallel.*
6. *Feel a lift in the body, as though creating space between the vertebrae.*
7. *The abdominal muscles, quadriceps and gluteus (buttocks) are used to maintain pelvic position.*

BE CAREFUL NOT TO:
☐ *rotate pelvis forward.*
☐ *push hips forward with straight legs and straight back.*
☐ *press chest forward by arching the back.*
☐ *work with weight on the heels.*

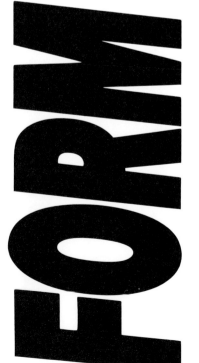

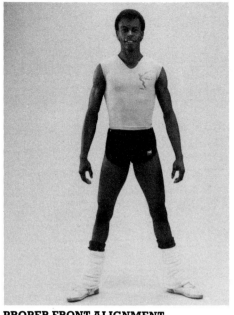

PROPER FRONT ALIGNMENT

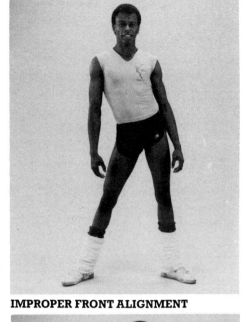

IMPROPER FRONT ALIGNMENT

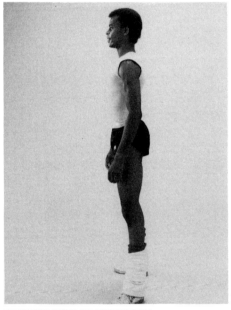

PROPER SIDE ALIGNMENT

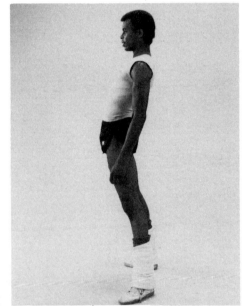

IMPROPER SIDE ALIGNMENT

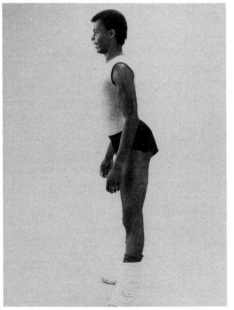

IMPROPER SIDE ALIGNMENT

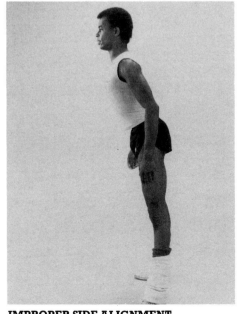

IMPROPER SIDE ALIGNMENT

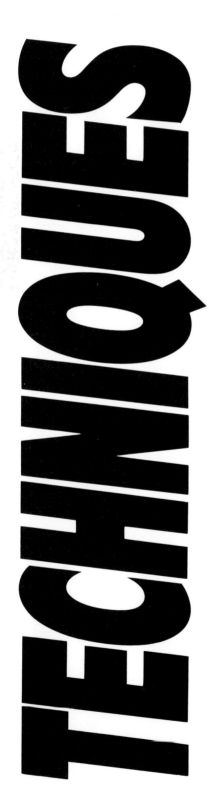

ARMS, SHOULDERS, CHEST AND BACK

1. Arms always work in front of the body's side plane, unless the exercise calls for a deliberate behind-the-back movement. This serves two purposes: it keeps the body weight on the toes and it helps prevent lower back hyperextension.

To test for proper arm position, (with arms in second position) move the arms all the way back past the side plane of the body, with eyes front. Slowly bring the arms forward until they can be seen via peripheral vision. Use the same technique to test for arm position above the head.

2. Arms always work with a stretch/reach feeling. The focus is always out.

3. Be careful of hyperextended (double-jointed) elbows. These types of arms should be placed in a position whereby the arm is straight, then reach from that point.

4. Use the arm muscles to create movement only and not torso impulses, rebounding or torso momentum. This is cheating or swinging.

5. When working the shoulders, keep them pressed down. This gives the neck a lengthened appearance. Lifting the shoulders creates unwanted tension in the upper back and neck.

6. When exercising the chest, you must create an isometric contraction as well as a mechanical contraction to produce sufficient work.

7. A high arm position works the upper chest, a medium arm position works the middle chest and a low arm position works the lower chest.

8. When exercising the back, the closer the arms remain to the body's side plane, the more efficient the work.

9. To avoid hyperextension of the lower back, care must be taken not to arch the back during standing back exercises.

WAIST

1. All the points of technique for stance and alignment, frontal and lateral, must be carefully observed when working on the waist.

2. Keep the arms in front of body's side plane.

3. The focus is 45 degrees high and not down or directly to the side. This limits hyper-lateral flexion of the spinal column.

4. Keep the head and torso in line, so that the head is an extension of the torso.

5. The shoulder line remains parallel to the front surface of the room.

6. The pelvis stays tucked back to lengthen the lower spine.

7. If a sway back creates a situation in which the subject cannot tuck the pelvis back while standing straight-legged, then a plie may be in order. This will give the pelvis room to tuck making the back less hyperextended.

PRE-CARDIO

Points of technique

1. Stance technique should be carefully observed, frontally and laterally.

2. The buttocks do not drop below knee level.

3. Control movements up and down – no bouncing.

4. Keep the arms in front of the body's side plane.

5. On fly-away exercise, a small contraction of the abdominals is present.

6. For any one-leg plie toe-touch, the extended arm goes to second position and stays at close as possible to parallel to the floor. For a toe-touch with both legs in plie, the arm goes either to the back or to the side. Never take the extended arm across the back.

7. On the upward part of big motions such as the fly-away and big toe touches, the body should rise into proper stance as described.

CARDIO

Points of technique

1. On landings, move through the foot – toe-to-metatarsal-to-heel. Reverse this order as the foot leaves the floor for jumps.

2. Use the leg muscles as shock absorbers. Use the plie, ie. bend the knees.

3. Keep the body weight forward.

4. Breathe. Most people do not have a problem taking air in, but they may hold it too long. Breathing must be continuous.

5. Improper shoes, improper foot positions, and hard workout surfaces will promote shin splints.

6. All cardio exercises start with a plie to initiate movement.

7. Keep arms in front of body's side plane.

ABDOMINALS

Points of technique

1. Lower back always maintains contact with the floor.

2. Top of pelvis should always be rotated back (pelvic tilt).

3. If an exercise is done with the extended legs, the legs go only as close to the floor as you can take them, while keeping the lower back on the floor.

4. Minimize the amount of torsion on the lower spine by keeping the angles of the shoulder line and pelvic line as close as possible to zero degrees.

5. The head remains in line with the torso or the chin is to the chest.

CAUTION! If you place your hands behind your head to pull the upper body when the abdominal muscles are tired this could cause problems by pulling on the cervical portion of the spine.

LEGS & BUTTOCKS

1. Doggie legs
body position as checked from the front:
a) Thigh on the supporting side stays as close as possible to perpendicular (vertical).
b) Angle of the pelvic line is as close as possible to parallel to the floor (horizontal).
c) Angle of the shoulder line remains as close as possible to horizontal.
d) Focus of the head is to the floor and the head stays in line with the torso.

Doggie legs
body position as checked from the side:
a) Arms (from shoulder to wrist) and leg (from buttock to knee) are perpendicular to the floor.
b) Abdominal muscles are contracted to tilt the pelvis back and keep lower back lengthened. Do not drop the lower back.
c) Focus on the raised leg is out and stretched, not up and lifted. The leg does not rise beyond parallel to the floor.
d) Angles between the floor surface, shoulder line and pelvic line should be as close as possible to zero degrees. Keep the back straight.
e) Head remains in line with the torso; maintain a feeling of lift and a lengthened body.

2. Chair and side leg
body position checked from front:
a) Lengthened feeling through the top of the head.
b) Maintain a feeling of lift in the body.
c) Belt line is perpendicular to the floor.
d) Shoulder line is square and parallel to the floor (except on side legs, resting on the elbow).

Chair and side leg
body position checked from side:
a) Shoulder line and pelvic line are parallel to front surface of the room, perpendicular to the floor.
b) Focus with the legs is out and stretched not up and lifted.
c) No weight is on the shoulder joints (except for side legs, resting on the elbow).

3. The knee goes out of line with the flex-and-stretch exercise.

4. The foot goes out of line with the kick-the-bum exercise.

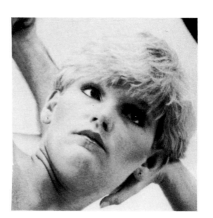

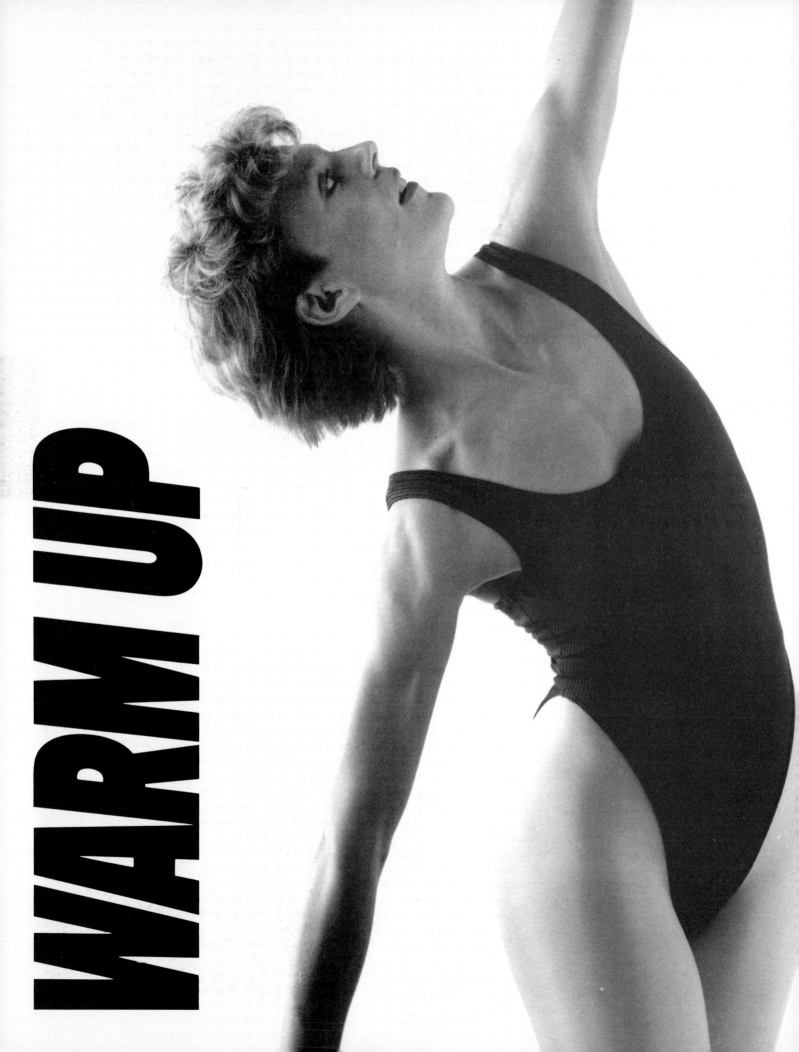

WARM UP

WARM-UP EXERCISES

SHOULDER LIFTS

Body Area:
Shoulders, trapezius.

Position:
Stand in second position, arms at sides.

Form:
Lift shoulders to your ears, then slowly lower them as far as you can, bending the legs at the same time and straightening them as your raise your shoulders again. Action should be smooth and controlled, not fast and jerky. The idea is to warm up slowly.

Variation:
This exercise can also be done rotating the shoulders backwards and forwards. As shoulders roll forward, feel the back open. Imagine an angered cobra spreading its hood. As the shoulders roll back, feel the chest area open and spread.

BREATHING ARMS

Body Area:
Lungs, diaphragm, arms, shoulders.

Position:
Stand in second position, with arms at sides.

Form:
Raise arms overhead while taking a deep breath. Lower the arms (under control) and exhale at the same tempo. Arms must be kept in front of the body's side plane. Remember that you are reaching with the arms as you lift them and relaxing them as they are lowered.

Variation:
Breathing arms with plie is performed by bending the legs at the same tempo that you raise the arms, then straightening the legs as you lower the arms.

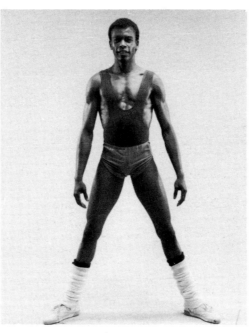
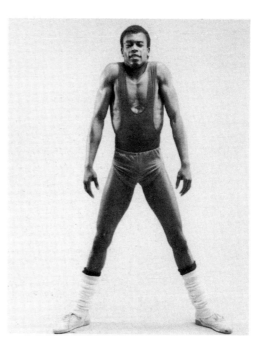
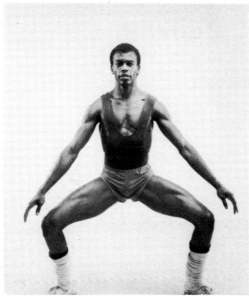

SHOULDER LIFTS

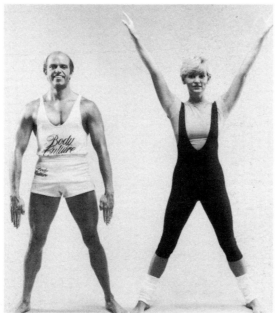
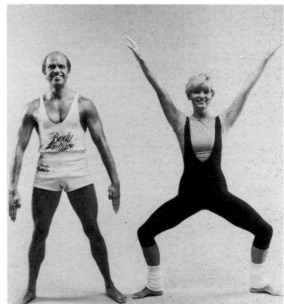

BREATHING ARMS

83

SIDE BENDS

Body Area:
Obliques, intercostals and serratus.

Position:
Stand in second position.

Form:
Lean body to one side while lifting the shoulder on the opposite side. Lower the shoulder as you bring the body back to center. Repeat on the other side, then repeat, without stopping in the center.
The action should be smooth and controlled, with consistent tempo. Remember, you are lifting one shoulder and stretching your side, not just falling over to one side with your upper body weight.

Variations:
The same can be done with both arms out to the sides. The exercises may be done with straight legs, or with plie.

WAIST ISOLATION

Body Area:
Quadriceps and obliques.

Position:
Stand in second position, arms at the sides.

Form:
Reach right arm to the right side of the room, bending slightly from the waist. On the second movement, bend the legs and reach both arms straight, toward the ceiling. On the third movement, reach the left arm to the left side of the room with straight legs. The fourth movement is like the second, with both arms straight up. Observe proper stance and plie techniques. Keep the movements slow and controlled.

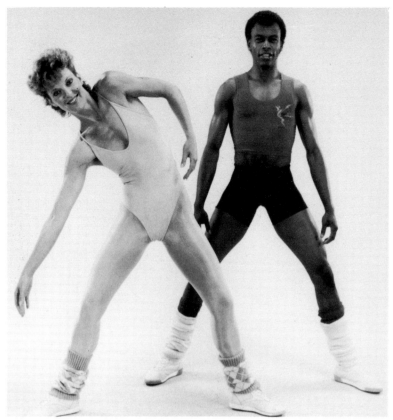

SIDE BENDS

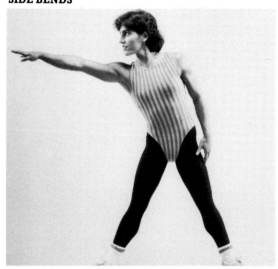

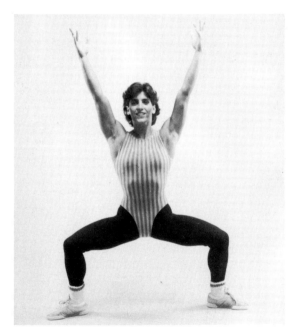

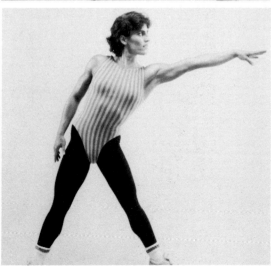

WAIST ISOLATION

MODERN DROP COMBO

Body Area:
Obliques, lower, middle and upper back.

Position:
Stand in second position, legs slightly bent.

Form:
Bend to the right, while feeling a stretch in the left side of the body. On the next movement, sweep the body toward the floor, feeling the shoulder blades separate to give a stretch across the upper back. The next movement is to take your body to the left, this time feeling a stretch in the right side. To complete the combination, move the body back to the right. Repeat the movements, beginning with a bend to the left. Observe the points of technique for stance and plie. The body remains relaxed and all movements should be slow and controlled. Do not drop the body.

ALTERNATE RIBCAGE STRETCH

Body Area:
Obliques, serratus, intercostals.

Position:
Stand in second position, arms above the head.

Form:
Stretch the right arm toward the ceiling while you relax the left arm. Hold for two seconds and then repeat, this time stretching the left arm and relaxing the right. Feel that you are trying to create space between the ribs on the side being stretched.

Variation:
An alternate ribcage stretch may be done with plie. As you stretch one side, the leg on that side bends slightly to accentuate the stretch. On the leg that is bent, be sure to keep the line of the thigh and the line of the foot in the same direction.

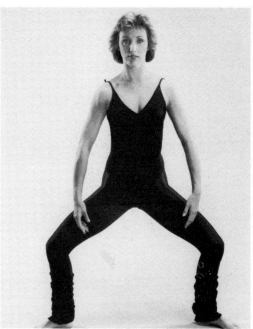
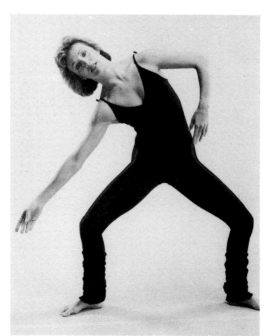
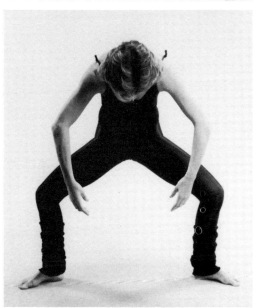

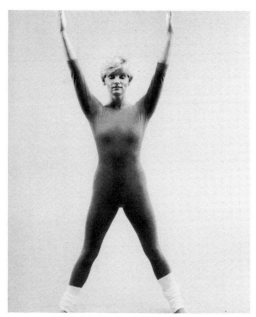
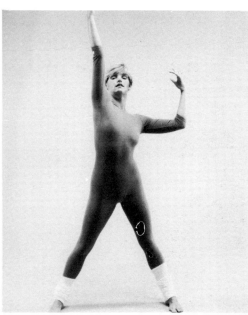
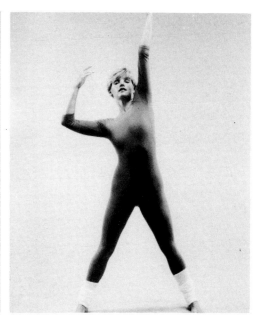

ALTERNATE RIBCAGE STRETCH

85

CONTRACTED FLYAWAY

Body Area:
Abdominals, quadriceps, arms, back.

Position:
Stand in second position, arms above the head with the palms facing forward.

Form:
Slowly bring the arms from their high position, through second position to a low position. At the same time, bend the legs slightly to plie, while tipping the top of the pelvis back and contracting the abdominal region. As the arms reach their low position, you should be at the depth of your plie and you should have achieved maximum contraction in the abdominal region. Return to original position.
Maintain proper stance, arm alignment and plie and check each time you return to original position.

PLIE AND STRETCH

Body Area:
Hamstrings.

Position:
Stand in second position with torso in maximum flex. The palms of the hands are on the floor, or as close to the floor as possible. The head is relaxed and follows the line of the torso.

Form:
Make certain the knees are lined up over the toes. Slowly bend the legs for four seconds to reach 90% bend, but don't allow the buttocks to go below knee level. Slowly return to original position, allowing four seconds to achieve straight legs. Feel a full stretch in the hamstrings. In this exercise, the upper body remains as relaxed as possible. The head stays in line with the torso.

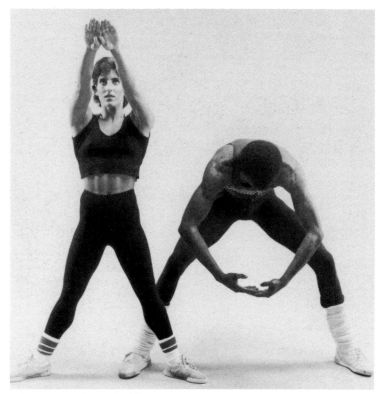

CONTRACTED FLYAWAY

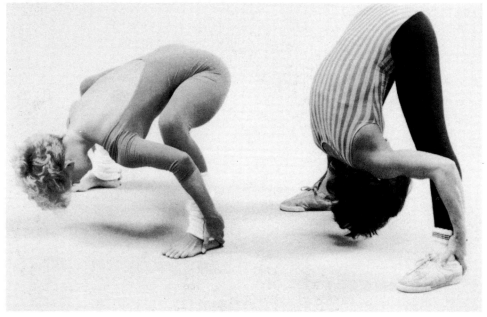

PLIE AND STRETCH

LONG LEG STRETCH

Body Area:
Hamstrings, obliques.

Position:
Same as "plie and stretch."

Form:
Grab the right lower leg with both hands and try to place the middle of the chest on the right thigh. Hold for 20 seconds, then release and relax the body back to starting position. Repeat on the other side.

Variation:
The long leg stretch with arm is performed the same way, except that the arm on the side being worked is stretched up toward the ceiling and you twist slightly.

Pointers:
If you cannot grab the ankle or get your chest to your thigh, grab the leg as low as you can and relax in that position.
Keep the toes pointed to the front of the room
Keep the pelvic line parallel to the floor to keep the hips square with respect to the floor.

ROLL UP (Transitional move)

Body Area:
Back.

Position:
Same as "plie and stretch."

Form:
This move brings the body from a low level to a high level. Start by bending the legs slightly and slowly lifting the upper body, with the back in a rounded position. You should feel the muscles in the lower back, then middle back and finally upper back and neck. Finish standing in second position with straight legs and perfect posture.

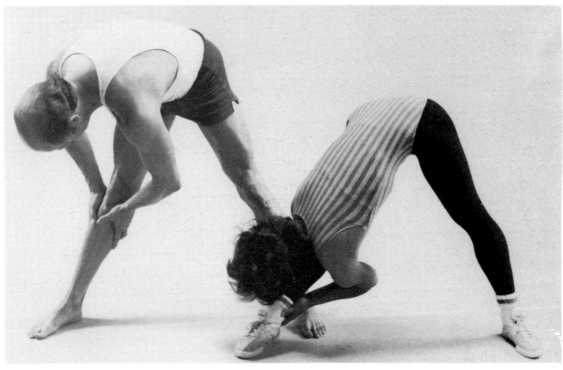

LONG LEG STRETCH

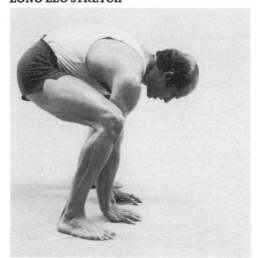

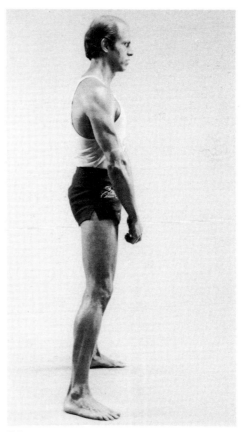

ROLL UP

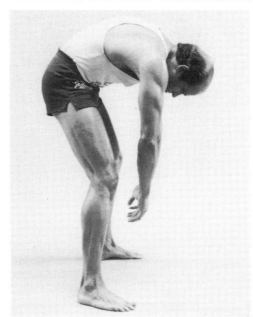

87

CONTRACT AND RELEASE

Body Area:
Abdominals.

Position:
Stand in second position, arms at the sides.

Form:
Slowly bring the arms from the sides to the front of the body, keeping them straight. At the same time, tip the top of the pelvis back as far as possible and contract the abdominal muscles. Slowly bring the body back to the original position.

Variation:
Contract and release with plie is performed by bending the legs so that the depth of the bend, the maximum arm stretch and maximum abdominal contraction all happen simultaneously.
As the arms stretch in front of you, feel a stretch across the upper back.

OPEN PRESS

Body Area:
Upper back, obliques, quadriceps and chest.

Position:
Stand in second position, arms bent so that the hands are in front of the chest.

Form:
Slowly rotate the torso to the left, at the same time bending the left knee and opening the arms, as if to open saloon doors. Return to the original position, rotating torso back to center, straightening the left leg and bringing the arms back to center. Repeat to the other side.
Arms must stay in front of the torso's side plane at full rotation. Don't rotate the body around too much. As the arms open, they should wind up parallel to the side surface of the room.

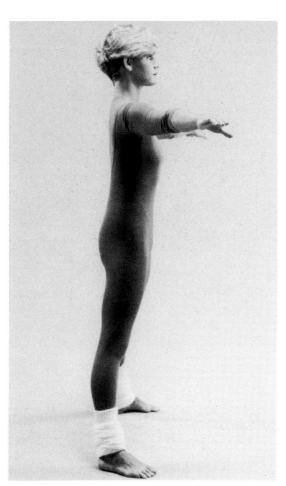 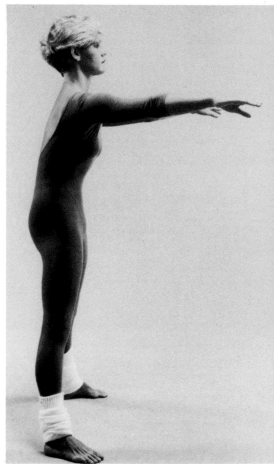

CONTRACT AND RELEASE

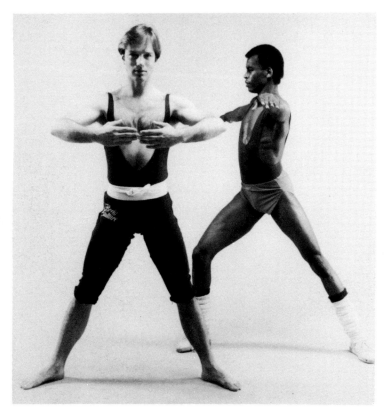

OPEN PRESS

FOUR-PART LUNGE SEQUENCE

Body Area:
Legs, calves, groin, hamstrings.

Position:
Assume the position in the first photo, the torso parallel to the floor, perpendicular to the front of the room. The buttocks level does not drop below the knees. The toe of the straight leg points to the side. On the opposite leg, the line from the knee to the heel is perpendicular to the floor, the heel down, and the line of the thigh matches the line of the foot.

Form:
Slowly transfer to the position in the next photo. Press the pelvis toward the floor, keeping the front heel down and the back leg straight.
Next, transfer to the position of photo three. For a more controlled stretch, you may decrease the distance between the feet at this point. Both legs are straight, with the pelvic line parallel to the floor. The back heel is aiming to touch the floor. In photo four, the body is in the center, with weight forward on the toes.
Repeat for the other side. When moving from one position to the next, make the transition slow and controlled.

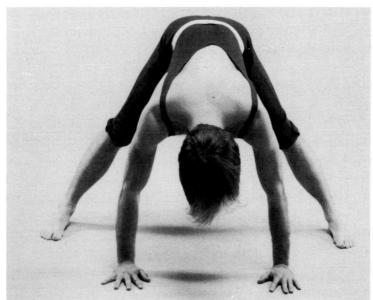

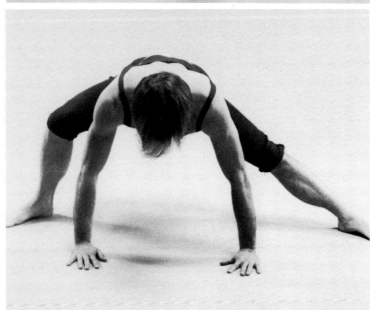

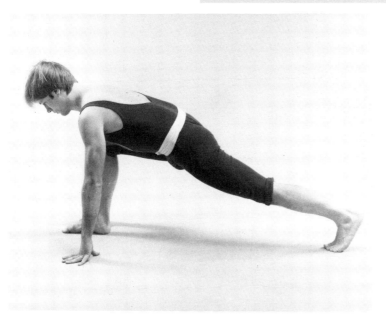

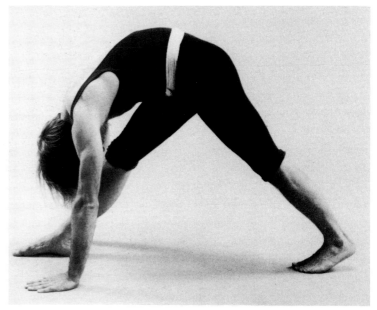

SHOULDERS

EXERCISES FOR ARMS, SHOULDERS CHEST AND BACK

SHOULDER CIRCLES

Body Area:
Chest, back and trapezius.

Position:
Stand in second position, arms at the sides.

Form:
Rotate the shoulders up in a circular motion. As you slowly bring the shoulders down, force them slightly forward to stretch the upper back. Repeat. On the upward rotation, the shoulders are pulled back to feel the stretch across the chest.

Variation:
This can be done with a plie following the movement of the shoulders. As the shoulders lower, the legs bend. As the shoulders lift, the legs straighten.

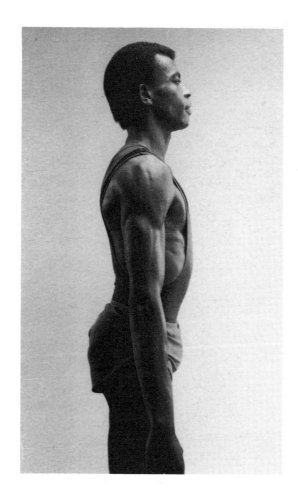

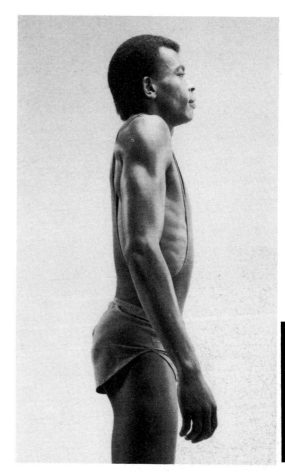

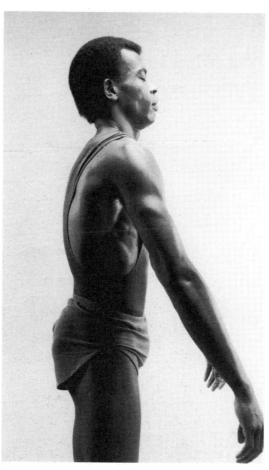

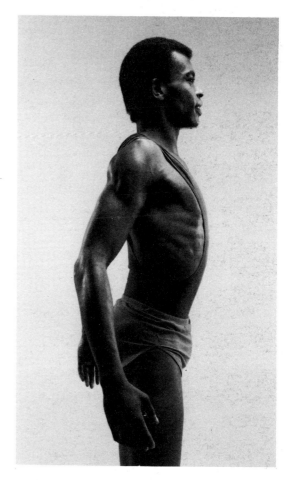

BIG BIRD

Body Area:
Middle and anterior deltoids (shoulders) and trapezius.

Position:
Stand in second position, arms relaxed at the sides.

Form:
Take the arms from a low to a high position, moving through second position. As the arms lift to the high position, feel that you are reaching. Stretch as you bring them back to the starting position, relaxing them for the last third of the downward movement. Remember to keep the arms in front of the body's side plane.

HAMMER FIST

Body Area:
Deltoids (shoulders).

Position:
Stand in second position with the arms down, palms facing the front of the thighs.

Form:
Start by lifting the arms straight from the thighs to a position over the head, reaching for a high point. Lower the arms under control, with deltoids flexed, in the same line, back to starting position. Be careful not to take the arms past the body's side plane and do not throw the arms into position.

Variation:
The same can be done with arms opening out to the sides. Stand in second position with arms stretched out in front of the chest. Feel the stretch across the upper back and slowly open the arms to the sides as the stretch transfers from the upper back to the chest. Return arms to front.

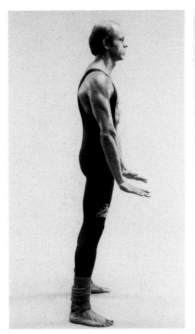 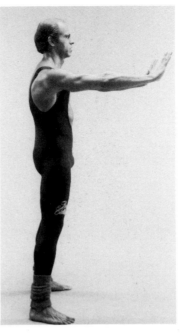 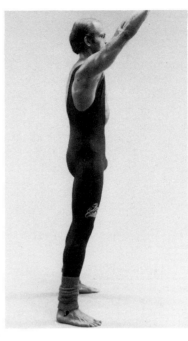

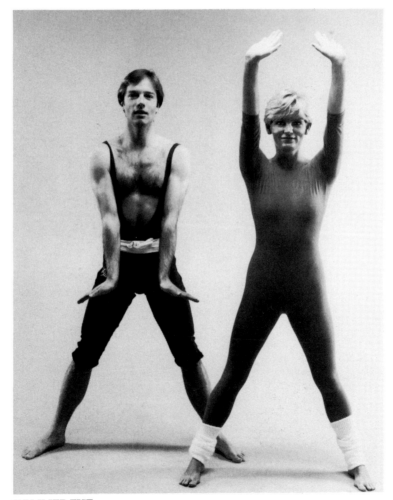

HAMMER FIST

92

SCISSORS

Body Area:
Deltoids and pectoralis (shoulders and chest).

Position:
Stand in second position, arms stretched in front of the chest.

Form:
The arms do a crossing action, imitating scissor blades. The action alternates with the right hand on top, then the left. The arms open only to shoulder width, then cross again. The action should be small and controlled.

Variations:
This movement can be done with the hands in front of the thighs, behind the buttocks or over the head. Each variation emphasizes a different shoulder area.

DELTOID PULSE (High)

Body Area:
Rear and middle deltoids (shoulders).

Position:
Stand in second position, with arms lifted above the head.

Form:
Maintaining correct body posture, press the arms backward about two inches, then release. Repeat. Don't hyperextend the lower back. The action should be small and precise. Keep the abdominal muscles contracted and keep the weight on the toes.
A variation, known as the deltoid pulse (side) can be done, pulsing the arms to the side.

DELTOID ROTATIONS

Body Area:
Deltoids (shoulders).

Position:
Stand in second position, arms out in second position.

Form:
Observe the body from the side. The fingertips move in small circles, each circle having about a four- or five-inch diameter. The arms can be circled to the back or front. The action should be small and controlled and a feeling of reach/stretch should be present.

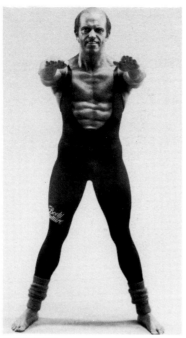
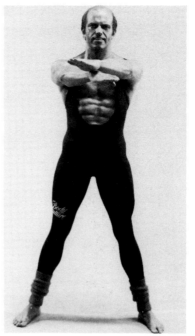

SCISSORS

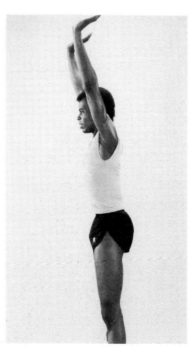

DELTOID PULSE

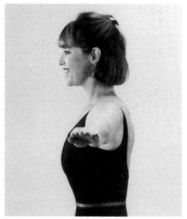
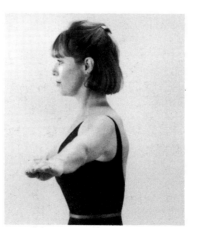

DELTOID ROTATIONS

ARMS

BICEP CURLS, Three Positions

Body Area:
Biceps.

Position:
Stand in second position, arms at the sides, elbows held in tightly against the waist and palms facing front. Make a fist with each hand.

Form:
From the starting position, slowly bring your fists up to the shoulders. Try to touch the knuckles of your hands to your shoulders, contracting the biceps. Keeping your elbows tight, return your fists to starting position as you relax the biceps.

Variations:
The same moves can be done with the arms stretched out to the sides, parallel to the floor, with the palms (fists) facing the ceiling or with the arms stretched to the front of the body. The actions should always be slow and controlled.

FOREARM SQUEEZES

Body Area:
Forearm flexors and extensors.

Position:
Stand in second position, stretching arms out to the side with palms facing the floor.

Form:
Slowly close your hands, contracting the forearm as tightly as you can. Open the hands and relax. Vary the exercise by performing it with the palms up, palms back and palms facing the front.

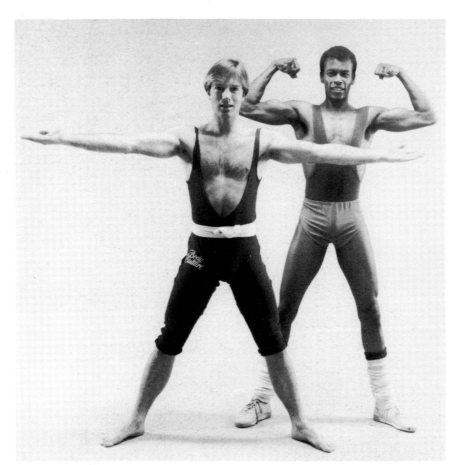

BICEP CURLS

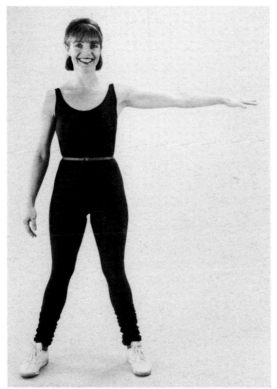

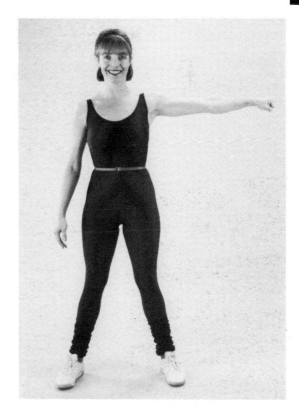

FOREARM SQUEEZES

WRIST CURL

Body Area:
Forearm flexors and extensors.

Position:
Stand in second position, arms outstretched at sides, with palms facing the floor. Make tight fists.

Form:
The focus of the exercise is on the flexor portion of the forearm. Slowly bring the knuckles down to the floor and, just as slowly, return to starting position.

Variations:
The exercise may be done with the the knuckles turning toward the front, the knuckles moving upwards (to work the extensors) or the knuckles reaching back.
Keep the fists tightly clenched for maximum benefits.

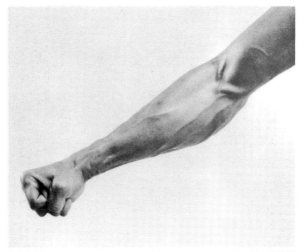

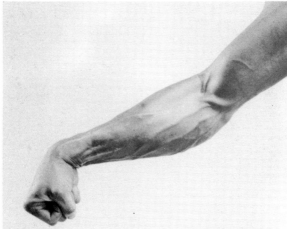

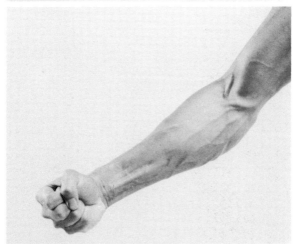

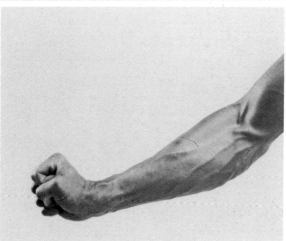

STANDING WEED PULL

Body Area:
Triceps (back of upper arm).

Position:
Stand in second position, arms bent, with wrists tucked in next to the waist and palms facing the ceiling (a karate pose).

Form:
Start by reaching arms over the head as if to grab hold of something. Spread the fingers. Imagine you are pulling something down. Return to original position. Next, extend the arms to the back with the palms facing down, contracting the triceps. Take care not to change the level of the elbows.
You must feel as if you are pushing something with the backs of your hands. Once your reach full extension, stretch the arms down and back. Return to original position. Do not arch the back when you achieve the full extension to the rear. On this particular exercise, the arms will go behind the body's side plane. This will be the case in all tricep work.

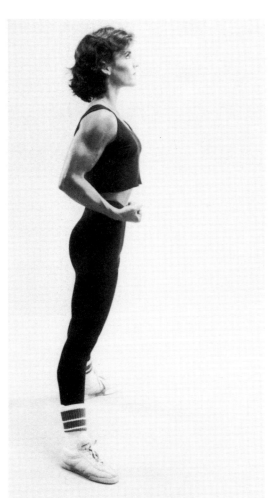
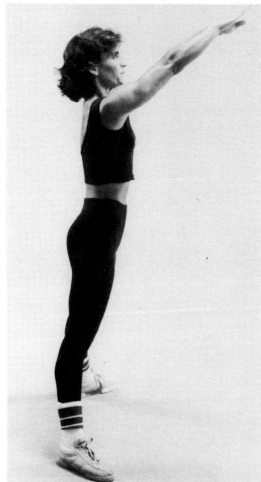
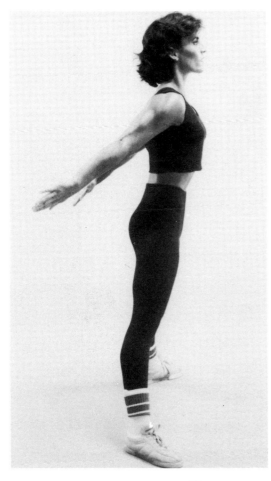

TRICEP EXTENSION

Body Area:
Triceps (back of upper arms).

Position:
Same as for standing weed pull, but the hands are formed into fists.

Form:
The tricep extension is the second half of the standing weed pull exercise. The arms extend to the rear, then return to the start position. Repeat.
This exercise should be done with the fists starting a little higher than in the previous exercise.

TRICEP EXTENSION PULSE

Body Area:
Triceps (back of upper arms).

Position:
Stand in second position, arms fully extended down the back, past the body's side plane, the palms facing front.

Form:
The action of this exercise is very small. The feeling from the start position is that of reaching down and back. The more reach, the more you will feel the triceps contract. Lift the back of the hands toward the ceiling and squeeze. Release back to original position. The distance moved is only about three to five inches. Take care not to hyperextend the lower back. The action is slow and controlled.

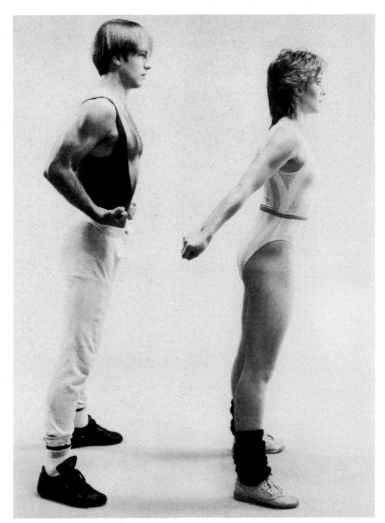

TRICEP EXTENSION

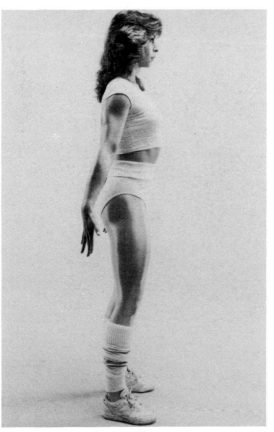
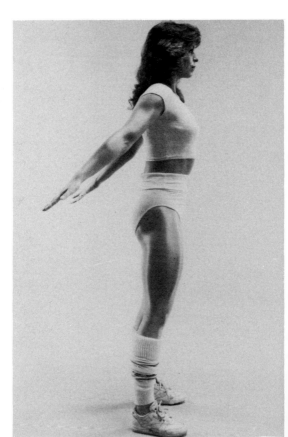

TRICEP EXTENSION PULSE

TRICEP ROTATION

Body Area:
Tricep.

Position:
Same as for the tricep extension pulse.

Form:
Achieve the same feeling of reaching, down and back. Slowly rotate the arm inward, flexing the tricep until the palms face the back. Return to the original position. Try to go for the full range of motion on both the turn in and the turn out. Take care not to arch the back. Movements are slow and controlled.

TRICEP EXTENSION CLAP

Body Area:
Triceps.

Position:
Same as tricep extension pulse, except that the palms face each other.

Form:
Reach down and back as in previous exercise. Clap the hands behind the buttocks.
Take care not to open the arms wide in preparation for the clap. The open position distance should be approximately shoulder width. Keep the arms as straight as possible. Not everyone will make contact on the clap.

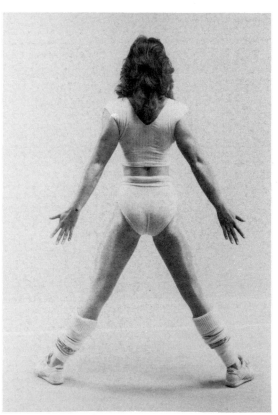 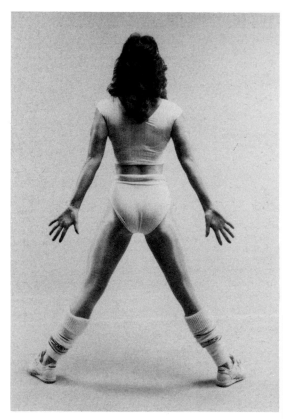

TRICEP ROTATION

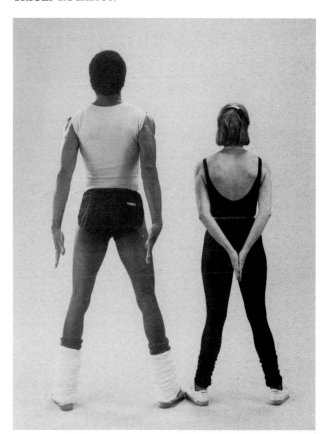

TRICEP EXENSION CLAP

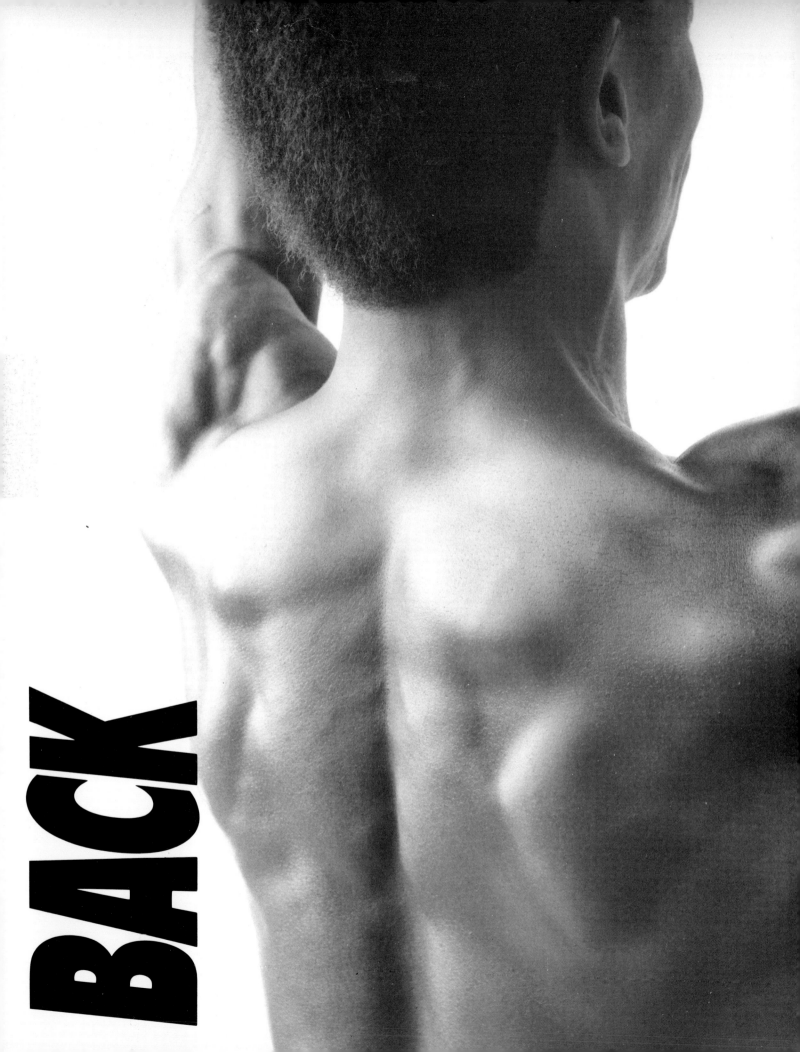

BACK

BLADE SQUEEZE

Body Area:
Rhomboids and trapezius (upper back), with secondary emphasis on the latissimus dorsi.

Position:
Stand in second position, arms outstretched to the sides, parallel to the floor.

Form:
The arms maintain a feeling of reach. Slowly squeeze the shoulder blades together, without disturbing the line of the arms. Release back to the original position. A variation may be done by isolating only one shoulder blade at a time.
Don't disturb the line of the arm. If the body were viewed from the top, the arms would be at an angle of about 175 degrees, even when the blades are squeezed together. Do not arch the back.

TABLE TOP BIG BIRD

Body Area:
Latissimus dorsi and trapezius. The lats are the large back muscles which, when developed, fan to the sides, giving the back width.

Position:
Second position, table top: to achieve the proper stance, begin with standing second position, arms at the sides. Keeping the arms at the sides, bend the legs slightly and bend the torso so that the back is parallel to the floor.

Form:
The arm action is like that of the standing big bird exercise. The arms travel through the second position, starting from the sides of the body and finish above the head.
In this position, the closer the arms stay in line with the body's side plane, the more the work will focus on the niddle to upper back. Make sure the level of the buttocks stays above knee level. The thigh stays in line with the toe. Plie technique notes must be carefully observed.

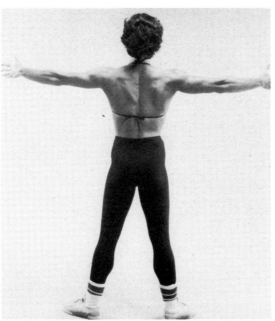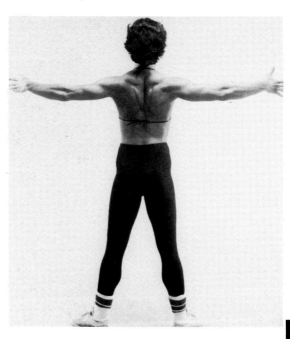

BLADE SQUEEZE

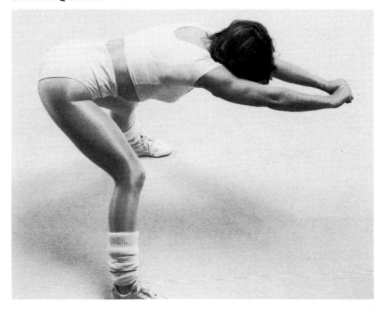

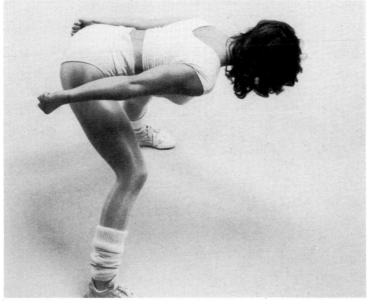

TABLE TOP BIG BIRD

TABLE TOP SECOND TO ELBOWS

Body Area:
Latissimus dorsi and trapezius.

Position:
Assume the table top position, with arms extended above the head in line with the torso. The palms face the floor, with the hands about six inches apart.

Form:
Use a bit of imagery for this exercise. Pretend you are taking hold of a broom handle with both hands. Pull the handle behind your neck, until you can't bend your arms any more. Return to starting position. Then pull once more, keeping the arms straight this time, until the arms come into line with the shoulders (second position for arms). Return to original position and repeat the sequence from the beginning.

Variations:
This exercise can be done with the arms extended toward the floor. Pull the imaginary broom handle toward the chest. The remaining portions of the exercise are the same, except that instead of the motion coming from above the head, it comes from the floor.
The actions should be smooth and controlled. The buttocks stay above knee level and the knees and toes in line with one another. Because of the body position, it becomes hard to arch the back. Therefore, on this variation, you may take the arms back behind the body's side plane. This is an exception to the rule.

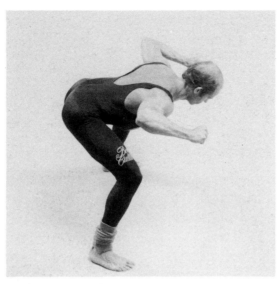
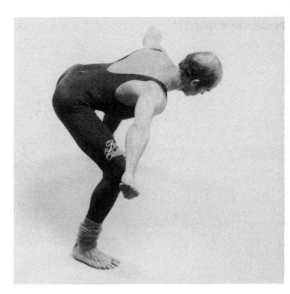
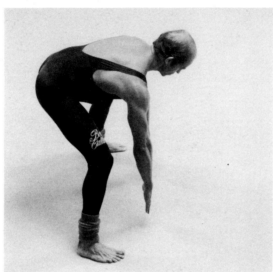
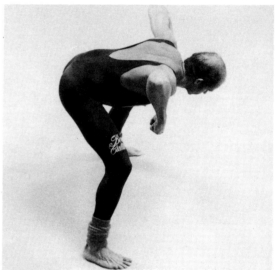

PULL DOWN ISOLATE

Body Area:
Latissimus dorsi.

Position:
Stand in second position, arms above head.

Form:
Imagine a piece of string is tied around your mid-section, just above the sternum. As you pull the arms down, bend them slightly until the elbows are in line with the shoulders. At that point, your objective is to try to flex your latissimus dorsi enough to break the imaginary string. Return to original position.
On the downward motion of the exercise, contract the lats on the sides of the body isometrically. The action of the arms is not enough to produce sufficient work for the lats.

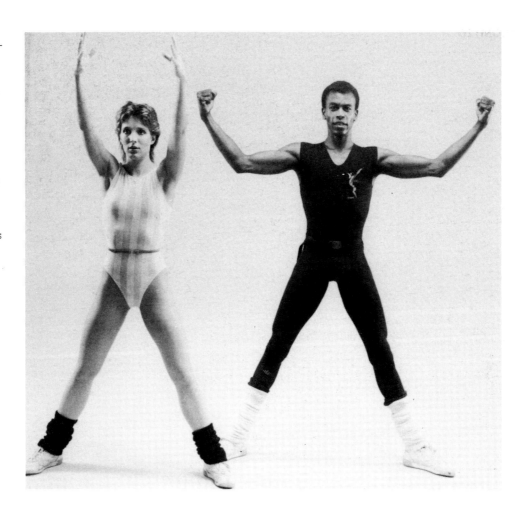

CHEST

PECK DECK

Body Area:
Pectoralis major (upper chest, or pectorals).

Position:
Stand in second position, with the legs slightly bent and the arms at 90 degrees in a muscleman pose.

Form:
Slowly bring the elbows and hands together, squeezing the upper portion of the chest. Do not allow the elbows to drop below the shoulder line. At the point of contraction, press the elbows together as tightly as possible. Release and return past the start position to get a nice stretch across the chest. Be sure not to arch the back.

Keep the line from the elbow to the shoulder parallel to the floor. In the closed position, focus your attention on the upper portion of the chest and squeeze the pectorals together. Don't hyperextend the lower back.

BENT ARM SCISSORS (Cable Squeeze)

Body Area:
Pectoralis major.

Position:
Stand in second position, arms stretched out to the sides, slightly bent at the elbows, palms facing the floor. Bend forward slightly.

Form:
Slowly pull the hands together, so they end up in front of the pelvis. During the descent, slowly squeeze the hands closed, so that at the bottom of the movement you achieve maximum contraction of the pectorals. Return to original position.

Variation:
This exercise can be done with the arms meeting opposite the sternum or over the head. The variations may all be done with straight arms. Keep the motions slow and controlled.

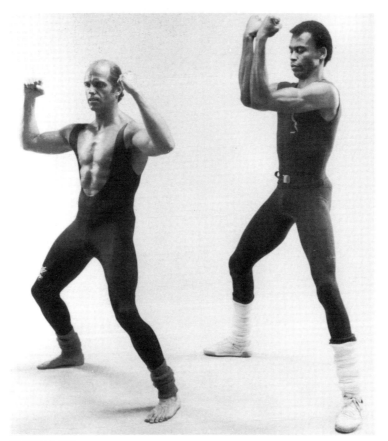

PECK DECK

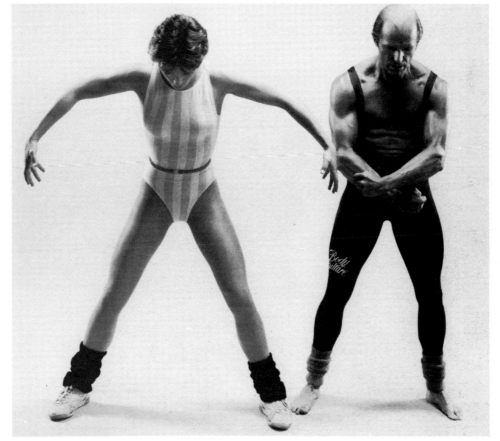

BEN ARM SCISSORS

WAIST

EXERCISES FOR THE WAIST

OVER TOP STRETCH

Body Area:
Obliques.

Position:
Stand in second position, left arm stretched out to the side and right arm relaxed, by your side.

Form:
Bend the body to the right and reach the left arm over your head at an angle 45 degrees to the floor. Direct the stretch up and out. Maximum stretch is achieved at 45 degrees. Return to the original position and repeat for the other side.
Observe proper stance techniques, laterally and frontally. Observe proper arm techniques and keep the torso lifted throughout the exercise.

SHOE LACE

Body Area:
Obliques.

Position:
Stand in second position, legs slightly bent, arms stretched out to the sides.

Form:
Slowly bend the body to the right, trying to create a 90-degree angle between your arm line and the floor. Your flexibility will determine your success. Slowly return to original position, then repeat for the opposite side.
This exercise must be done very slowly and smoothly. It is the only exercise that will reach the lower (inferior) fibers of the oblique muscles. It will also create lateral flexion of the lower spine. If this creates back pain, see your chiropractor. Take it easy and keep it controlled.

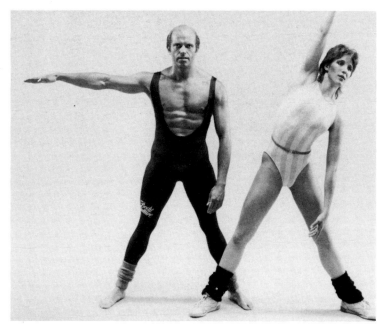

OVER TOP STRETCH

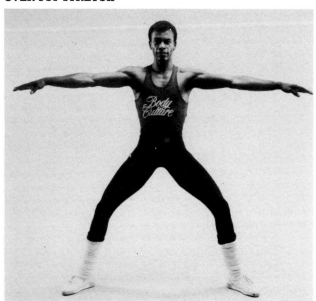

SHOE LACE

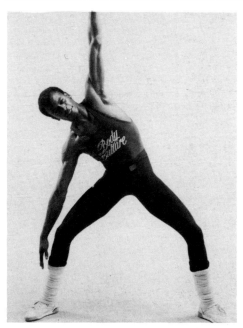

PULLING ROPE

Body Area:
Obliques.

Position:
Stand in second position, arms above the head, as if you were about to pull the rope in a bell tower.

Form:
Slowly imitate the action of pulling the rope down. Make a lateral bend as you pull your hands down toward one side of the body. At the instant you reach maximum body bend, the hands should reach the bottom of their downward pull. Reverse the motions to return to center and repeat for the other side.
With this exercise, the tendency is to lean back with the upper body as the arms finish their downward pull. This causes hyperextension of the lower back. The bend is lateral only. The shoulder line must be parallel to the front of the room so there is no torsion in the spine.

BOW AND ARROW

Body Area:
Obliques.

Position:
Same as pulling rope exercise, above.

Form:
The image for this is that you are shooting an arrow at the sun. As you draw the bowstring back, the body does a side bend. These happen simultaneously – at the maximum pull on the bowstring, you should be at the depth of the side bend. Slowly return to the original position, following the same path of movement. Repeat for the other side.
Don't arch your back at the depth of the side bend. The movement should remain lateral in nature.

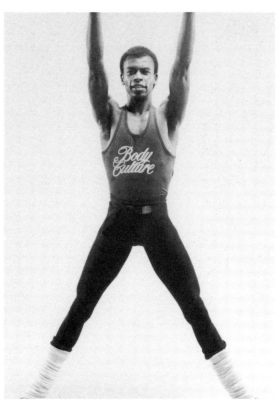
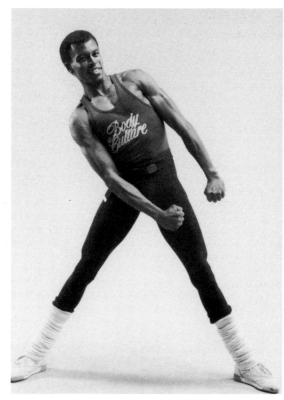

PULLING ROPE

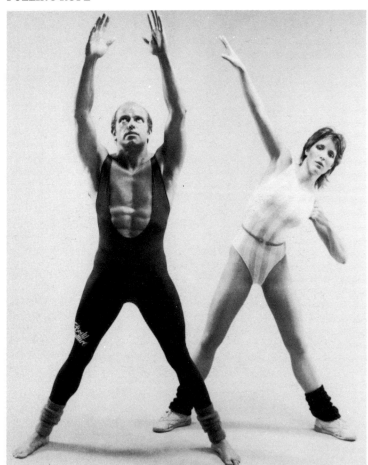

BOW AND ARROW

108

MONKEY PULL

Body Area:
Obliques.

Position:
Stand in second position, arms stretched out low, diagonally. The palms face the rear wall.

Form:
Bend the body slowly to the right, stretching the right arm to the side until it is parallel to the floor. At the same time, the left arm bends so that the left hand is in front of the chest. Return to the starting position following the same line of motion. Repeat for the left side.
Keep the arms in front of the body's side plane. Do not create and angle between the belt line and the floor. Once you get the feel of this exercise, you may pass through the start position instead of stopping in the center.

TRUNK TWIST

Body Area:
Obliques.

Position:
Stand in second position with the fingertips on the shoulders, elbows out.

Form:
Slowly rotate the body as far as possible, so that you face the side of the room. Keeping the movement slow and controlled, return to the starting position. Inhale at the start of the exercise and exhale as you twist. As the body returns to starting position, inhale once again. Repeat for the other side.
Twist the torso to its maximum range of motion, but do it slowly and with control.

Variations:
This may be done with legs straight or bent and with the arms in the muscleman pose or stretched out to the sides.

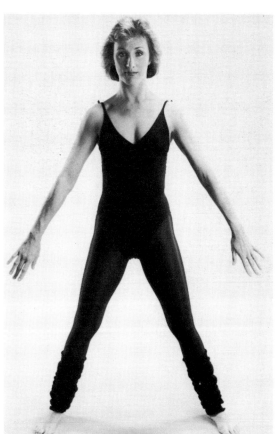 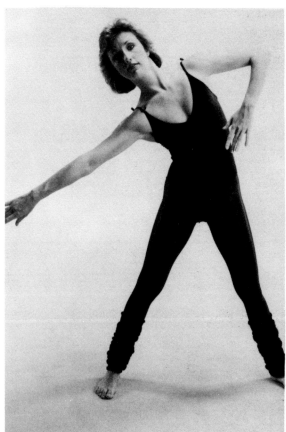

MONKEY PULL

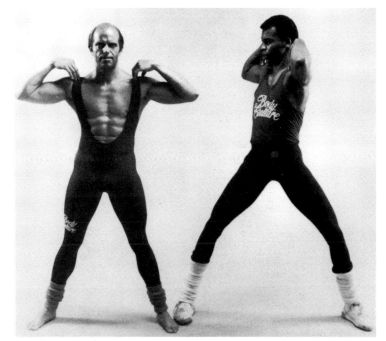

TRUNK TWIST

CARDIO

PRE-CARDIO EXERCISES

FLY-AWAYS

Body Areas:
Lower back, abdominals, intercostals, quadriceps, deltoids.

Position:
Stand in second position, arms above the head.

Form:
Take a deep breath and slowly bend the knees and bend at the waist until the torso is parallel to the floor. As the body descends, exhale slowly and let the arms travel through second position to a final position similar to a bear-hug. This posture helps to create a contracted abdominal section, which serves to protect the back. Feel the stretch across the back. Return to the original position by reversing the action and inhaling on the way up.
Both the downward and upward movements should be smooth and controlled. The body should not drop down too fast and the buttocks must not go below knee level. Keep the head and torso in the same line. Observe proper plie technique and keep the arms in front of the body's side plane.

FLY-AWAYS WITH KNEES UP

Body Areas:
Lower back, abdominals, intercostals, quadriceps, deltoids.

Position:
Stand in second position, arms also in second position.

Form:
This is done the same way as the regular fly-away, except that as you return to starting position, you lift one knee up with the upper body. The opposite elbow crosses over to meet the lifted knee, while the other arm is stretched out to the side. Return the raised foot to the floor as you go back down into the hugging posture. Repeat, using the opposite leg and elbow.
Remember to breathe in as you start, exhale on the way down and inhale on the way up. Don't let the raised knee cross the body. Bring the elbow across to touch the inside of the knee, thus preventing torsion in the lower back.

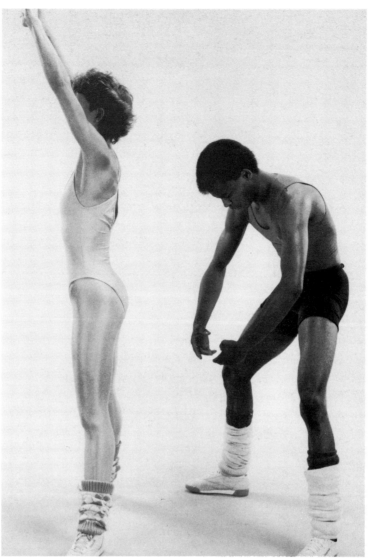

FLY-AWAYS

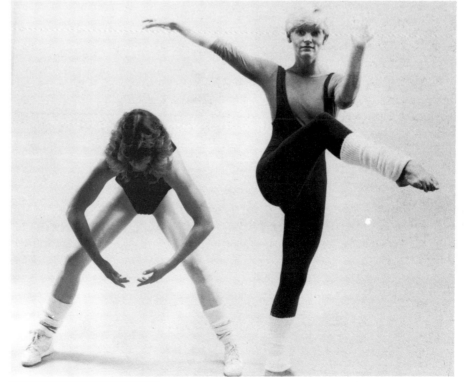

FLY-AWAYS WITH KNEES UP

111

SIDE-TO-SIDE TOE TOUCH WITH LUNGE

Body Areas:
Quadriceps, gluteus maximus, hamstrings, calves, deltoids.

Position:
Stand with feet apart, one and a half times shoulder width. The body is over in the lunge position as in the previous exercise. The left hand goes to right toe, with the right arm extended to the side.

Form:
Transfer the body from right to left as you change arm positions and touch the toes alternately. Repeat. Keep the head in line with the torso. The buttocks do not fall below knee level. The extended arm should reach to the side, not to the back as in the two previous exercises.

KNEE UP

Body Areas:
Psoas, abdominal muscles, quadriceps.

Position:
Stand with feet about six inches apart, with arms in second position.

Form:
Lift the knee as close as possible to the chest. The foot leaves the floor in the following sequence: heel, metatarsal, toes. This sequence is reversed as the foot returns to the floor. Repeat, using the other leg. Maintain an erect body posture, with the knee coming up to the chest, not the chest dropping to meet the knee. Observe proper stance and arm placement.

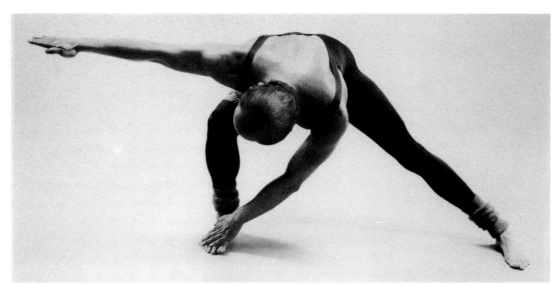

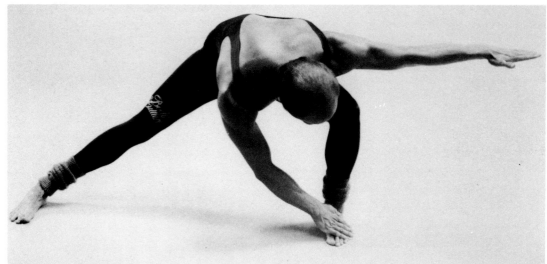

SIDE-TO-SIDE TOE TOUCH WITH LUNGE

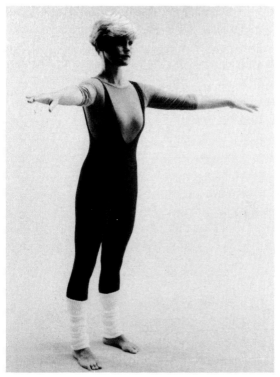
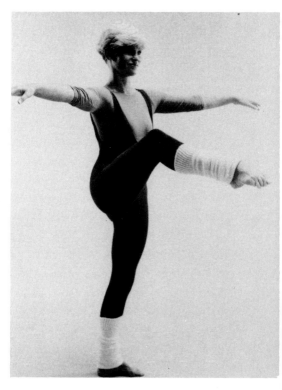

KNEE UP

TOE TOUCH WITH PLIE

Body Areas:
Quadriceps, deltoids, lower back, gluteus maximus (buttocks).

Position:
Stand in second position, arms over head, shoulder width apart.

Form:
Slowly bend the legs and bring the body down, so that the right hand touches the left toe and the left hand stretches to the back. Slowly bring the body back to the original position. Repeat, using the left hand to touch the right toe.
Keep movements controlled, up and down, and keep the head in line with the torso. Keep the spine, from head to tailbone, parallel to the floor, perpendicular to the front surface of the room. Don't let the buttocks fall below knee level.

TOE TOUCH WITH LUNGE

Body Areas:
Quadriceps, deltoids, lower back, gluteus maximus (buttocks).

Position:
Stand in second position, the feet apart, about one and a half times shoulder width, and the arms over the head, shoulder width apart.

Form:
This starts out the same as the previous exercise, with the exception of the legs. Only one leg is bent as the body lunges down – eg. if the left leg bends, the right hand crosses to touch the left toe. Return to original position and repeat to the other side.

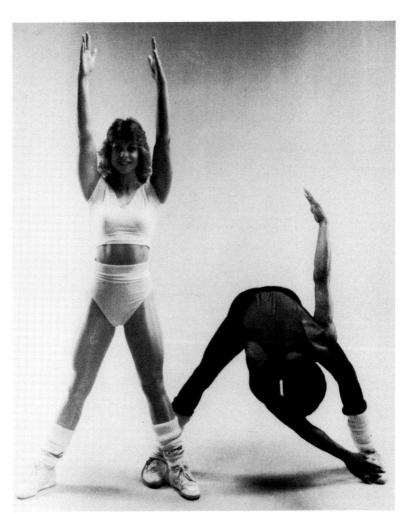

TOE TOUCH WITH PLIE

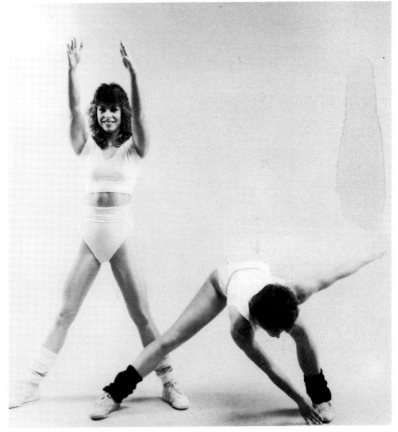

TOE TOUCH WITH LUNGE

EXERCISES FOR CARDIO

DOUBLE KNEE UP

Body Areas:
Psoas, quadriceps, calves.

Position:
Start with feet together, arms outstretched over the head in a "V".

Form:
Spring from both feet onto the right foot. At the same time, bring the left knee up to the chest (or as high as you can get it) and the right elbow down to touch the inside of the left knee. Without changing the upper body position (torso and arms) bring the left foot down to touch the floor, then back up to the high position.
Spring back to two feet, this time returning the arms to the "V" position above the head. Repeat, lifting the right knee to meet the left elbow. The working knee comes up twice before changing sides.

Variation:
This exercise may also be done bringing the knee up only once before the change.
Keep the body weight forward and be sure that the elbow touches the inside of the knee gently. Try not to take the high knee across the body, but rather endeavor to keep the line of the thigh perpendicular to the front surface of the room.

RUNNING (KNEE HIGH)

Body Area:
Psoas, quadriceps, calves.

Position:
Start with the feet together, arms at your sides.

Form:
Jump from the right foot to the left foot, bringing the right knee up to the chest. Repeat, alternating left and right knee up.

Variation:
This exercise may be done lifting the heels to kick the buttocks instead of raising the knees to the chest (Running Kick Bum). You may also do alternating sets of the two.
Keep the body weight forward, as this prevents the pelvis from tipping forward and arching the back. Take care not to slam the ball of the foot down with either of these exercises, as it may lead to shin splints.

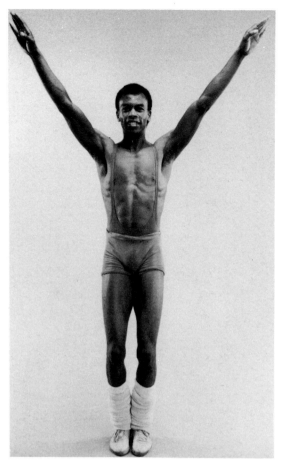 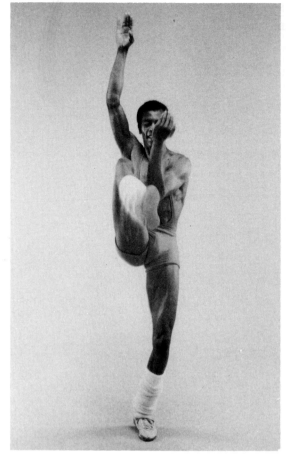

DOUBLE KNEE UP

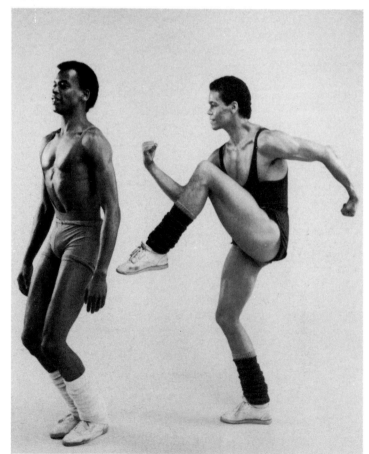

RUNNING (KNEE HIGH)

STRIDE JUMPS

Body Areas:
Calves, abductors and adductors (inner and outer leg), deltoids and trapezius (shoulders).

Position:
Start with the feet together, arms at your sides, palms facing the back wall.

Form:
Jump and place feet in second position. At the same time, the arms travel out from a low position to a high position, over the head. The arms reach the top position at the same time the feet land. Jump from second position back to the starting position, with the arms coming down to the sides as the feet hit the ground again. Repeat.
Keep the arms reaching on both the upward and downward movement.

PENDULUM

Body Areas:
Deltoids, quadriceps, calves.

Position:
Stand on the right leg, with left leg off the floor and extended to the side at a 45-degree angle. The left hand gently rests on the left thigh, while the right arm is extended above the head at a 45-degree angle.

Form:
Spring from the right leg onto the left leg. The right leg leaves the floor to assume the 45-degree angle extended position. The arms change position in the same time and tempo. Keep the arms straight and stretched. Ensure that the high arm remains in front of the body's side plane.

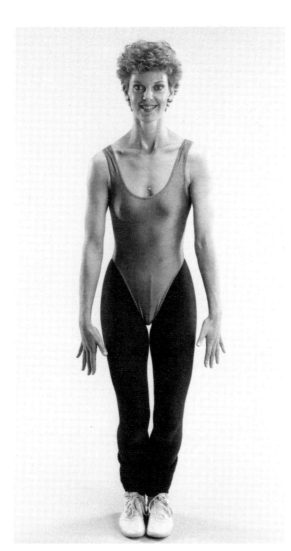
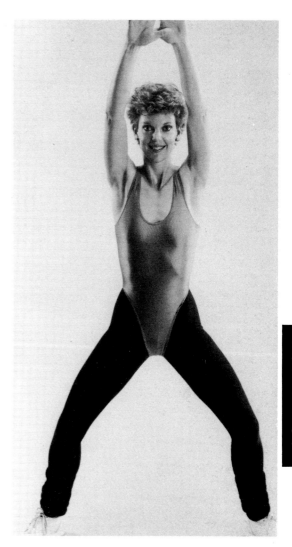

STRIDE JUMPS

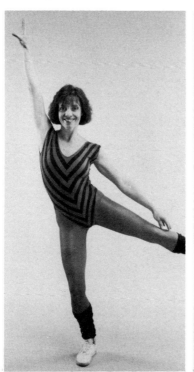
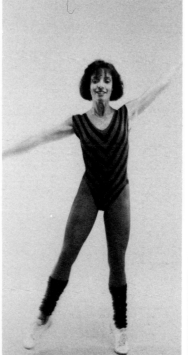
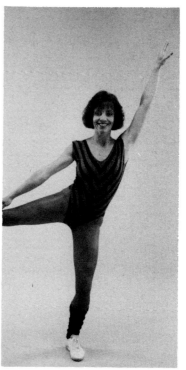

PENDULUM

115

SKI JUMPS

Body Areas:
Quadriceps, calves, hamstrings.

Position:
Feet together, legs slightly bent. The arms are bent and at your sides, as if holding ski poles.

Form:
Keeping the feet and the knees close together, jump to the left, landing on both feet with legs bent. Jump to the right, keeping both feet and knees close together. Repeat.
Be sure to keep the knees over the toes. The line of the thigh and the line of the foot should follow the same direction.

CROSSES (SMALL KICKS)

Body Area:
Calves, hamstrings, quadriceps, sartorius (inner thigh).

Position:
Start with the right foot on the floor and cross the left leg in front of the right, keeping the left foot off the floor. The left arm is in a low position, crossed in back of the body. The right arm is in a low position, crossed in front of the body.

Form:
Hop twice on the right foot, then change legs and arms and hop twice on the left foot. Repeat. Once you become proficient at this exercise, it can be done with single hops instead of double hops.

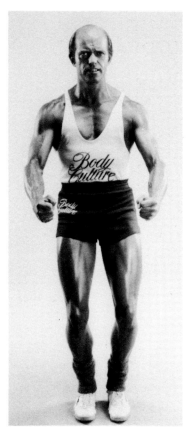 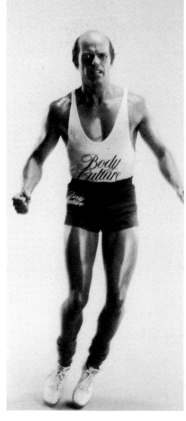 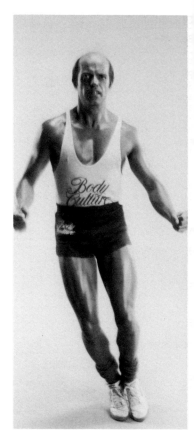

SKI JUMPS

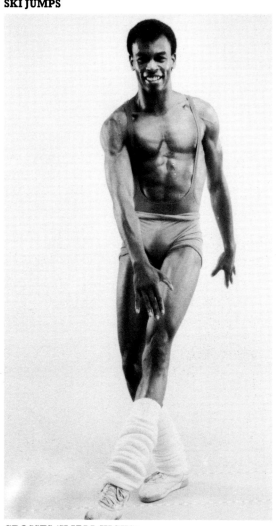 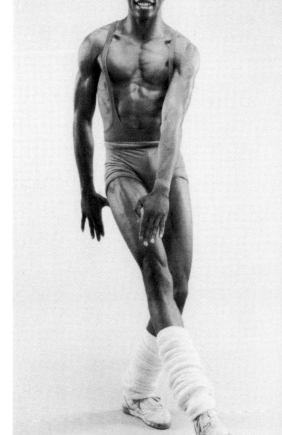

CROSSES (SMALL KICKS)

116

CROSSED TOE TOUCHES

Body Areas:
Calves, quadriceps, hamstrings, psoas and abdominals.

Position:
Stand on the right foot. Lift the left foot and position it in front of the thigh, about one foot away. The right hand touches the left foot, while the left hand is extended over the head.

Form:
This is very similar to the preceding exercise. Hop twice on the right leg, then change to the left leg, changing arm and foot positions simultaneously. This exercise may also be done with the raised foot in the back.

MOON WALK

Body Areas:
Deltoids, calves, quadriceps, hamstrings.

Position:
Start with right foot in front, left foot back; left arm in front, right arm back.

Form:
Simply jump and exchange the position of the feet and position of the arms at the same time. Return to the original position in the same manner. Be sure all the extremities move simultaneously and finish simultaneously. This is for body balance.

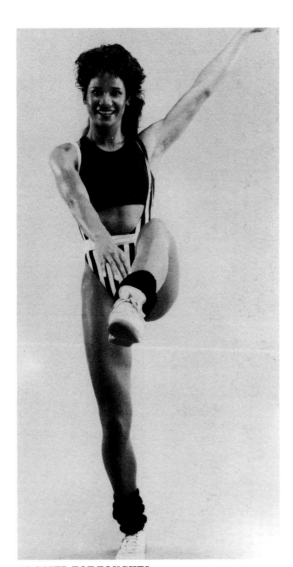

CROSSED TOE TOUCHES

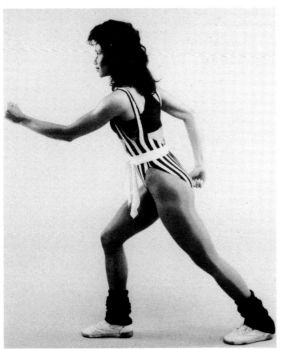
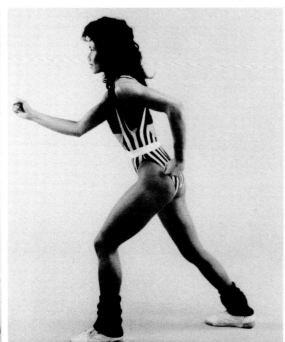

MOON WALK

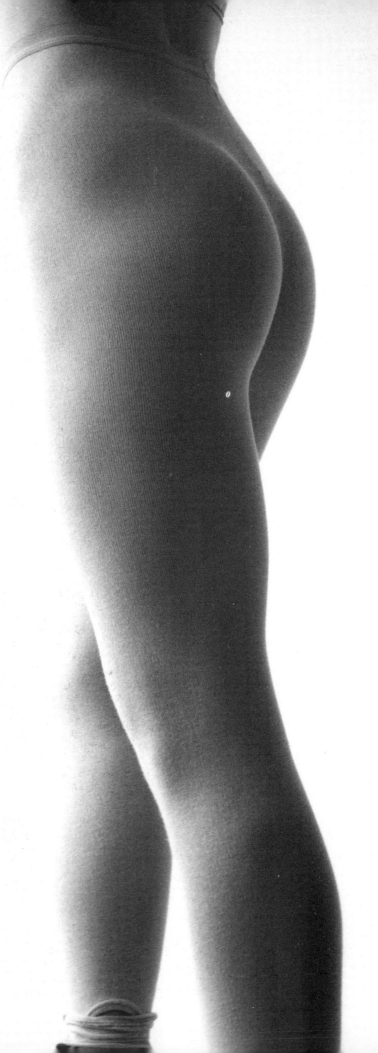

LEGS

EXERCISES FOR THE LEGS AND BUTTOCKS

SIDE LEG RAISE

Body Area:
Tensor fasia latae, gluteus medius and minimus (side hip and buttocks).

Position:
Lie on your side with the upper body supported on the elbow. The body is lifted; the spine is long. The line from the shoulder to the elbow should be perpendicular to the floor. The legs are stretched along the floor. Feel that you are trying to touch the far wall with your toes.

Form:
Lift the top foot away from the bottom foot, six to eight inches. Return the leg almost to the original position, maintaining a space of about one inch between the feet. Repeat.

Variations:
This exercise may also be done with a flex-and-stretch action or a kick-the-bum action.
The raised leg must feel constantly stretched, as if you want to make it longer than the other.

TURN IN, TURN OUT

Body Areas:
All gluteal muscles, quadriceps, tensor fasia latae.

Position:
Same as in side leg raise, but the foot is flexed.

Form:
Keeping the toe and knee in the same line, rotate the leg outward as much as possible and hold for three seconds.
Next, rotate the leg inward as much as possible and hold for three seconds. Repeat.
Be sure to squeeze buttocks together in the outward rotated position. The pelvic line must remain perpendicular to the floor.

Variation:
You may place the legs in a turned-out position and execute the flex-and-stretch movement.

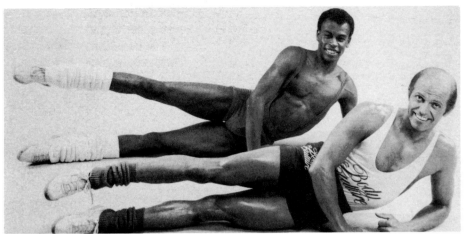

SIDE LEG RAISE

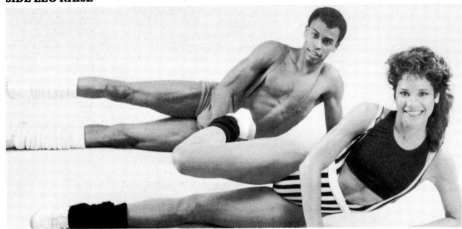

VARIATION

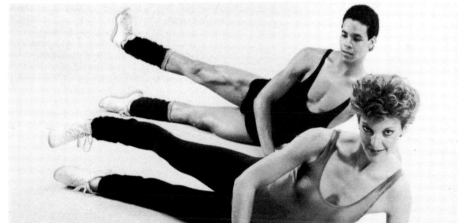

TURN IN, TURN OUT

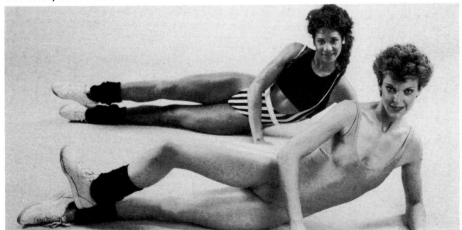

VARIATION

119

SITTING CHAIR LEGS

Body Areas:
Gluteus minimus and medius.

Position:
Lie on your side, with the legs pulled up in a sitting position.

Form:
Extend the top leg to reach toward the front surface of the room. It is parallel to the floor. Raise the leg slowly to an angle of 45 degrees, taking four seconds to do so. Slowly return the leg to original position and repeat. Keep the pelvic line and shoulder line perpendicular to the floor. Maintain a feeling of reach with the raised leg.

Variation:
You may hold the leg at 45 degrees and perform the flex-and-stretch action or the kick-the-bum action.

ADDUCTOR RAISE

Body Area:
Adductor brevis, magnus and pectinous (inner thigh).

Position:
Same as in side leg raise, except that the top leg is bent with the knee up and the foot placed about three inches in front of the knee of the bottom leg.

Form:
Flex the foot of the bottom leg. Using the inside of the thigh, slowly lift the bottom leg toward the ceiling and hold for three seconds. Maintain a feeling of reach. Return to original position, just off the floor. The inside of the working thigh faces the ceiling.

Variation:
This may be done with the flex-and-stretch action. The leg must be in the elevated position before you start to flex and stretch and the spacing between the foot and knee is about six inches.

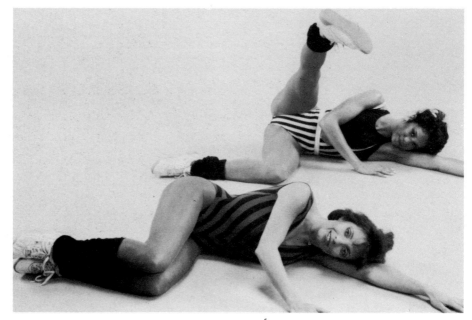

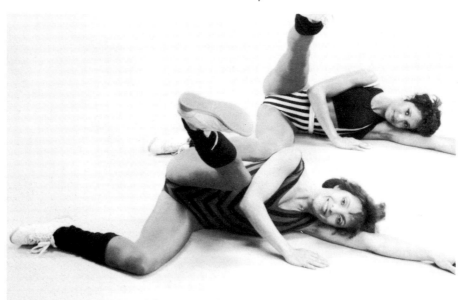

SITTING CHAIR LEGS

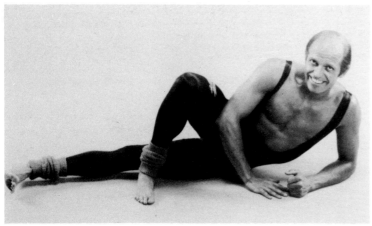
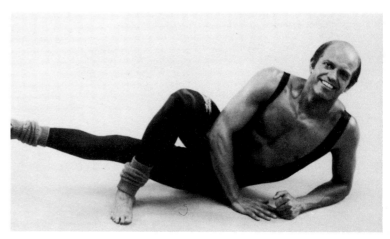

ADDUCTOR RAISE

HAMSTRING TUCKS

Body Area:
Hamstrings.

Position:
Lie on the floor on your back, knees bent and feet together. Raise hips and lower back off the floor.

Form:
Slowly press the hips toward the ceiling, pulling the heels toward the buttocks. Hold for three seconds, then return to original position.

Variations:
The exercise may be done with knees and feet approximately eight inches apart, or with one leg off the floor. If you choose a one-legged version, you may use the flex-and-stretch action, flexing as the hips drop and stretching as the hips rise. A more advanced version can be tried by supporting the body on the hands (with the upper body off the floor) and using all the variations.
Don't arch your back. The focus is on the hamstrings, so keep the buttocks relaxed. In the advanced version, keep the buttocks lower or on the same level as the knees.

BUM TUCKS

Body Area:
Gluteus maximus.

Position:
Same as for hamstring tucks.

Form:
The movement is basically the same as for hamstring tucks, except that when you press the hips to the ceiling, you squeeze the buttocks muscles together. As you come back to the original position, relax the buttocks muscles.
Don't arch the back; keep the lower back as straight as possible. The focus of this exercise is on the buttocks, not the hamstrings. For the advanced version of this exercise, see hamstring tucks.

Variations:
Optional foot and knee placements:
– feet together, knees apart
– feet apart, knees apart
– feet apart, knees together
– feet together, knees apart
– feet apart, knees apart, pulsing knees together
– feet together, knees apart, pulsing knees apart.

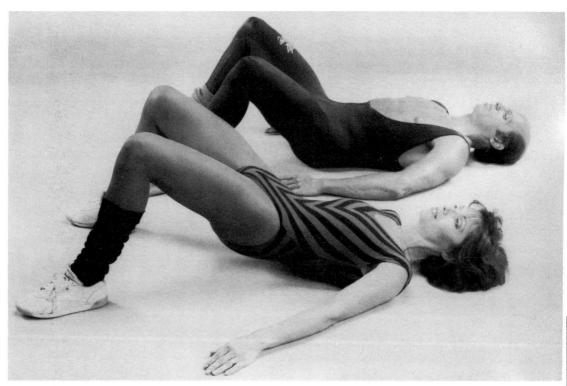

HAMSTRING TUCKS

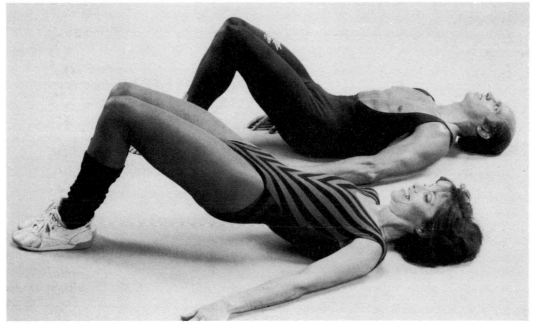

BUM TUCKS

DOGGIE LEG

Body Area:
Gluteus maximus.

Position:
The body is supported on all fours, as shown.

Form:
Slowly lift the knee as high to the side as you can, without disturbing the placement of the body. Hold for three seconds, then return to the original position. Observe all the points of technique for the doggie leg.

Variation:
This exercise may be done with an extension of the lower leg as the knee reaches its highest point. Keep the leg extended for two seconds, retract it, and return to original position.

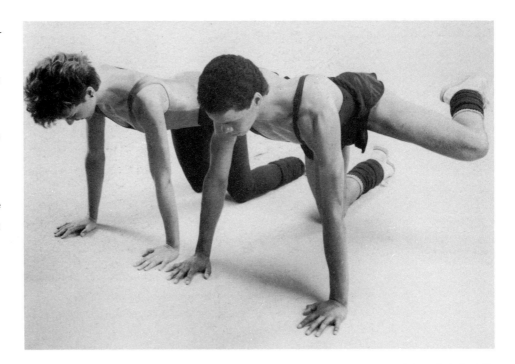

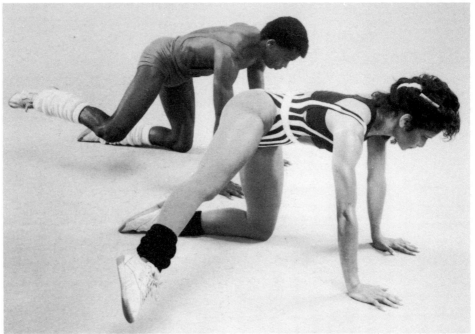

VARIATION

DOGGIE LEG REAR PULSE

Body Area:
Hamstrings.

Position:
On all fours, as in previous exercise.

Form:
Slowly extend the right leg to the back, making sure that the leg is reaching long and parallel to the floor, with the knee facing down. Lift the leg about five inches and hold for three seconds. Return to the original position. Remember that even though you are lifting the leg, the primary feeling is one of stretch toward the rear wall.

Variations:
This exercise can be done turned in (medial rotation) or turned out (lateral rotation). The leg may be held at its highest point and then rotated continuously. The exercise may be done with a flex-and-stretch action or the kick-the-bum action. It may also be done with the leg bent at 90 degrees, pulsing the heel to the ceiling.

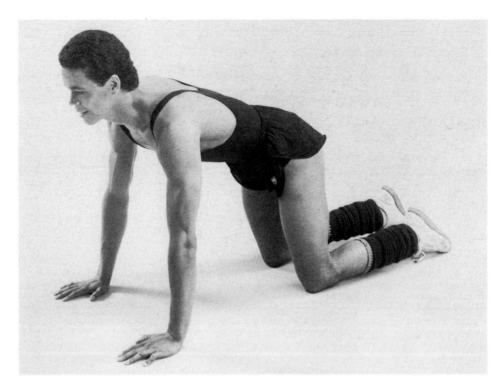

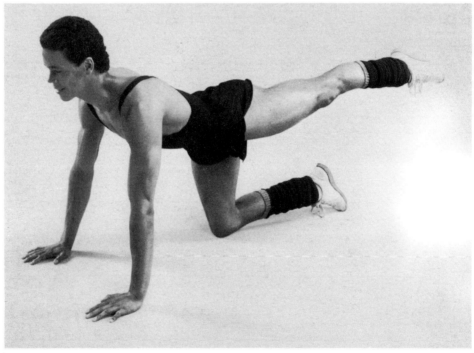

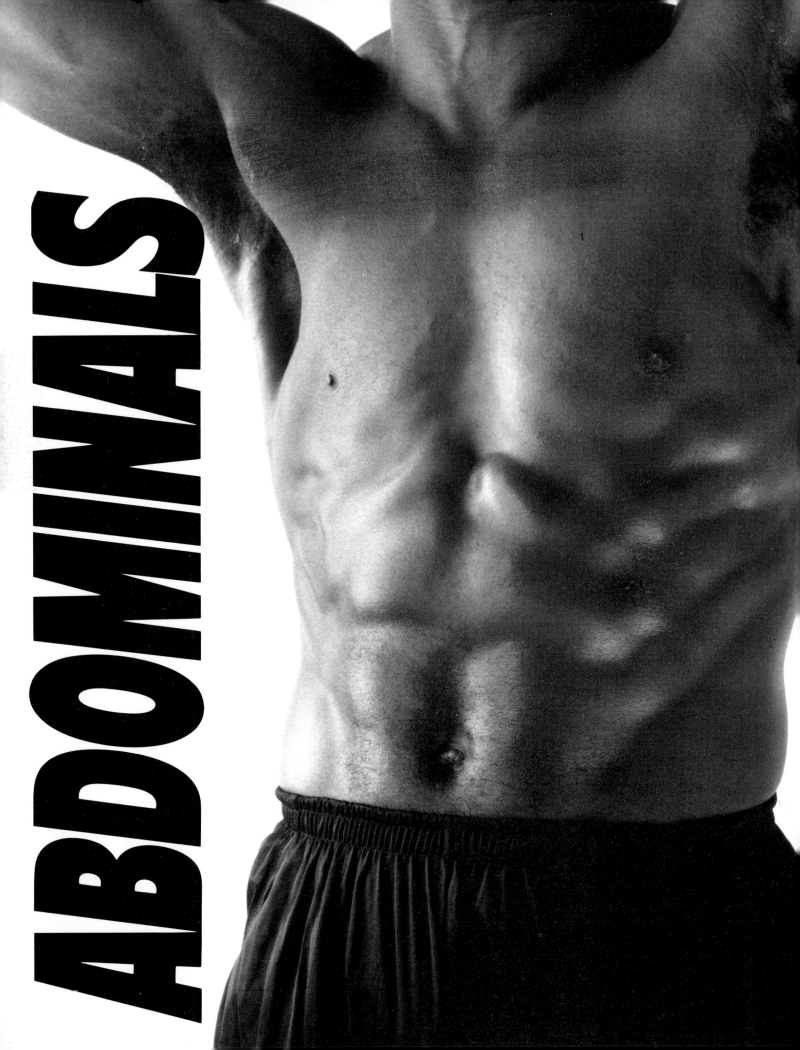

ABDOMINALS

EXERCISES FOR THE ABDOMINAL MUSCLES

LEG RAISE – 45 DEGREES AND 90 DEGREES

Body Area:
Lower abdominals.

Position:
Lie face-up on the floor, with the hands under your buttocks, palms down. Flex the head and upper body forward so that the lower back is pressed into the floor.

Form:
Bring the knees toward the chest at 90 degrees and extend the lower leg so that the toes point to the ceiling. Lower the legs slowly, until the angle is about 45 degrees, and return to original position. Concentrate on contracting the lower abdominals. If you don't have the flexibility in your hamstrings to reach a 90 degree angle, leave the legs slightly bent to protect the lower back. Observe all points of technique for abdominal work.

SITTING 15-DEGREE CRUNCH

Body Area:
Lower and middle abdominals.

Starting position:
Sit with the feet flat on the floor, with bent legs. The arms reach toward the front. The upper body leans to a 45-degree position. Be sure that the abdominal muscles stay contracted and that the back is not arched. Use the image of trying to press your navel to your back.

Form:
Extend one leg and gently lift about eight inches (about 15 degrees). Hold for one second, then return to original position.
Perform a predetermined number of repetitions with one leg, then repeat with the other leg.
You will feel some work in the quadriceps, which are used to extend the leg. Concentrate on using your lower abdominals only.

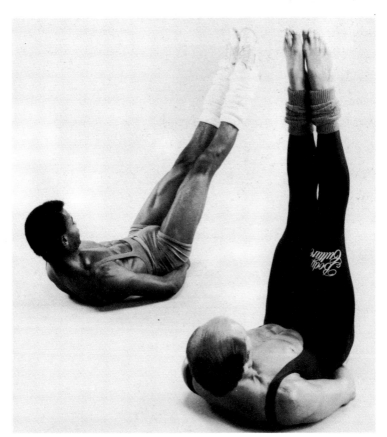

LEG RAISE

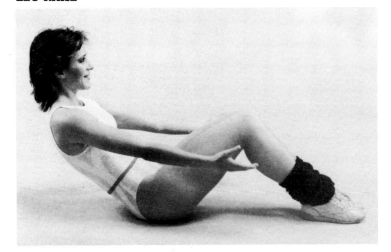

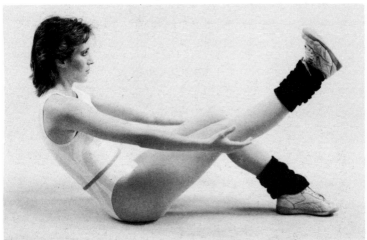

SITTING 15-DEGREE CRUNCH

125

BICYCLE

Body Area:
Lower abdominals, obliques.

Position:
Lie supine on the floor with fingertips at the side of the head. The right knee is pulled in to the chest and is in contact with the left elbow. The left leg is extended at approximately a 45-degree angle to the floor.

Form:
Keep the back on the floor and slowly bring the left knee to the chest while extending the right leg. At the same time, the right elbow reaches to meet the left knee. Return to original position and repeat. The elbow reaches to make contact with the inside of the knee.

Variations:
At the advanced level, the bent leg may be extended as it touches the opposite elbow. The lower part of that leg extends up, so that both legs are now straight.

BIG WALKS

Body Area:
Upper and middle abdominals.

Position:
Lie supine on the floor, hands (palms down) under the buttocks and legs bent at a 90-degree angle to the floor. Flex the neck and head forward.

Form:
Lower one leg until it is at a 45-degree angle to the floor. Slowly bring it back to the original position, while the other leg drops to the 45-degree position. The legs move simultaneously, as if walking on the ceiling.
Keep your back firmly on the floor. The leg closest to the floor does not fall so low as to release the back. Maintain a feeling of reach with the legs.

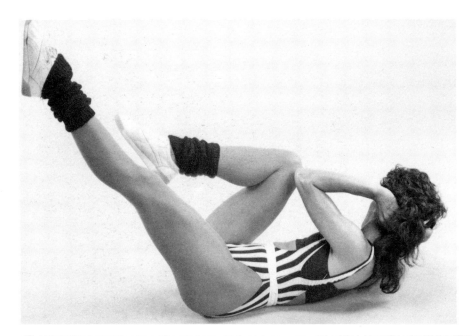

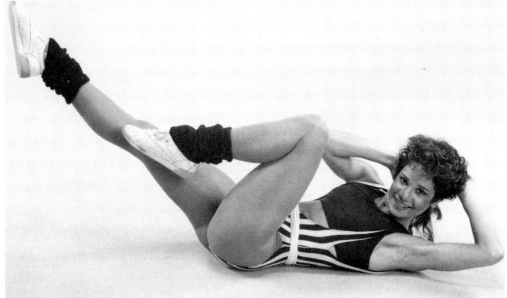

BICYCLE

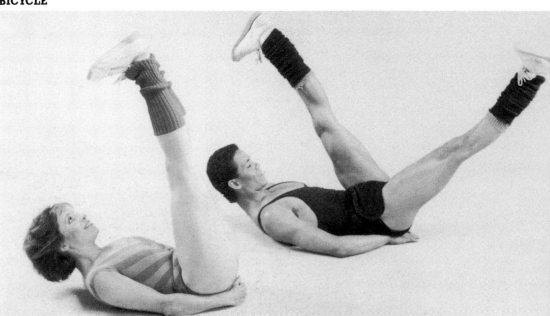

BIG WALKS

CRUNCH

Body Area:
Upper abdominals.

Position:
Lie on your back, legs open in second position. The back is pressed to the floor and the arms reach through the legs.

Form:
From this position, flex the neck and head forward, bringing the upper body as high as possible. Hold for three seconds, then release about two inches. Repeat.

Variations:
This may be done with the legs slightly bent to protect the back. By bending the legs, the pelvis has room to tip back.
The exercise may also be done with both legs together and pointed toward the ceiling. The arms reach to the front surface of the room, outside the legs.
A third variation may be done with the feet flat on the floor, knees bent and the palms of the hands gently rubbing the tops of the kneecaps. Always hold the contracted position for three seconds and only release two inches before contracting again. This keeps the work in the abdominal area.

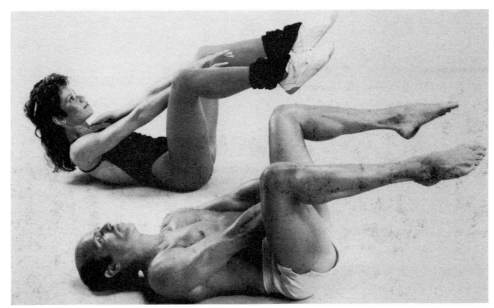

CRUNCH

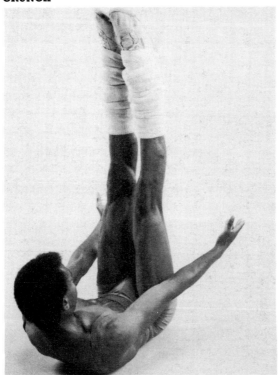

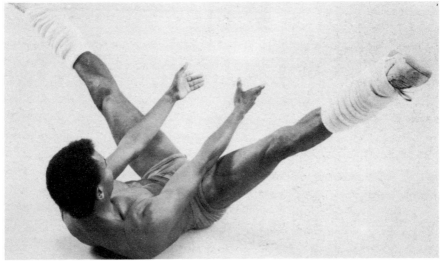

VARIATION

127

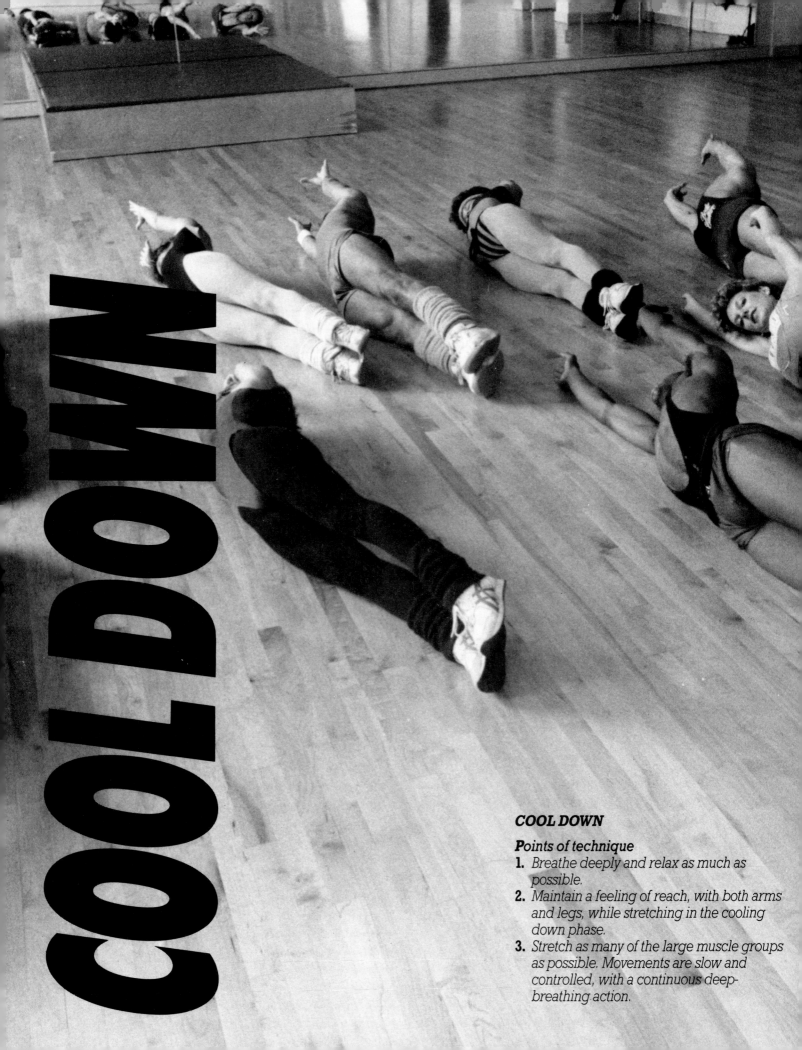

COOL DOWN

COOL DOWN

Points of technique

1. *Breathe deeply and relax as much as possible.*
2. *Maintain a feeling of reach, with both arms and legs, while stretching in the cooling down phase.*
3. *Stretch as many of the large muscle groups as possible. Movements are slow and controlled, with a continuous deep-breathing action.*

EXERCISE FOR COOLING DOWN

FULL STRETCH (RECOVERY)

Body Area:
Arms, Back, Stomach, Lungs

Position:
Lie supine on the floor with the arms above the head in the same line as the torso.

Form:
Roll onto your right side and place the body in a fully arched position. Return body to centre, then roll to the left and repeat the arch. Roll the body back to the centre. Next, stretch the right arm and left leg while relaxing the left arm and right leg. Continue stretching opposite limbs.

BREATHING FOCUS

Body Area:
Lungs

Position:
Lie supine on the floor, arms at your sides. The legs are bent, the feet flat on the floor and the knees pointed at the ceiling.

Form:
Breathe in through the nose – four seconds for complete inhalation – expanding the abdominal region so that the navel rises. Don't arch the back. Exhale through the mouth, again timing four seconds, and relaxing the abdomen so that the navel falls.

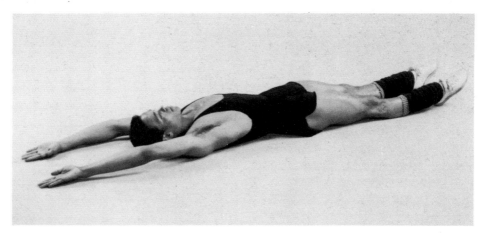

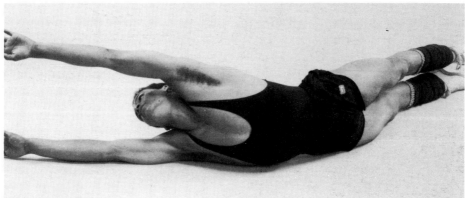

FULL STRETCH

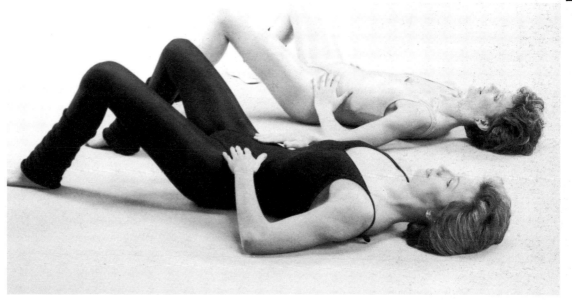

BREATHING FOCUS

CONTRACT AND LIFT

Body Area:
Arms, Lungs, Back

Position:
Sit on the floor with the legs together, torso erect. The arms are in the second position.

Form:
Take a deep breath, then release the air from your lungs as the arms stretch to the front. Collapse the diaphragm by contracting the abdominal section, rounding the lower back toward the back wall. Take a deep breath as you return to original position.

BREATHING

Position:
Sit with the legs bent, the bottoms of the feet together. The arms are outstretched to the sides. The upper body is tall and lifted.

Form:
Lift the arms over the head while taking a deep breath. Relax the arms back to the original position while expelling the air. Take four seconds to raise the arms up and four seconds to bring them back down.

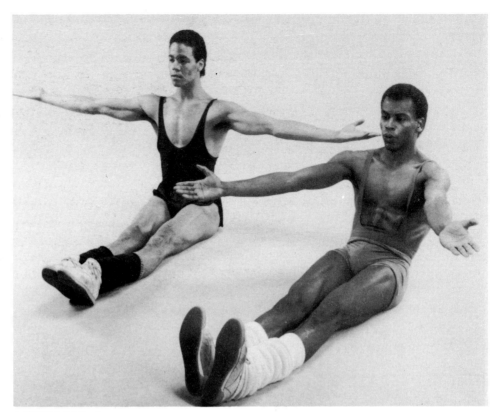

CONTRACT AND LIFT

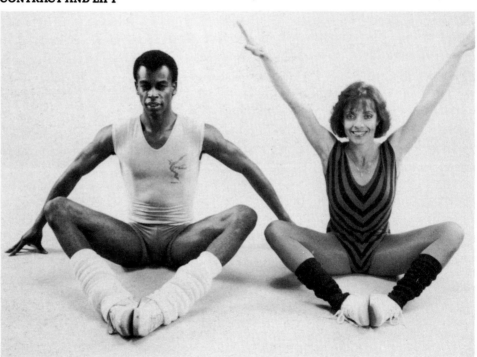

BREATHING

KNEE TO CHEST (HAMSTRING STRETCH)

Body Area:
Hamstrings and gluteal muscles.

Position:
Same as for breathing focus.

Form:
Slowly bring the right knee straight into the chest with both hands. Grab the right leg below the knee (the more flexible you are, the closer your grip to the foot). Flex the foot and slowly extend the leg. Hold for four seconds, then slowly return to original position. Repeat with the other leg. Keep it slow and controlled and remember to breathe deeply the entire time.

SECOND POSITION FLOOR STRETCH

Body Area:
Groin and hamstring stretch.

Position:
Sit on the floor with the legs in a straddle position.

Form:
Gently relax the body down over the right leg, head to knee. Hold for 20 seconds. Slowly move the head between the legs and hold for 20 seconds. Move head to left knee and hold for 20 seconds. Return to centre and hold for another 20 seconds. Extend the torso and lift the arms while taking a deep breath. Exhale and lower the arms in the same tempo as the exhalation.

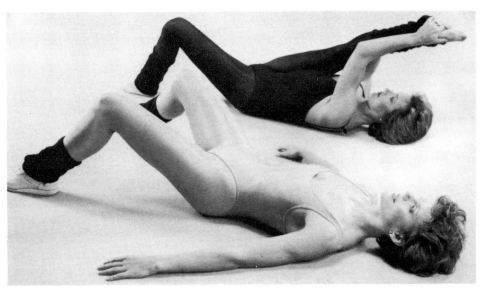

KNEE TO CHEST (HAMSTRING STRETCH)

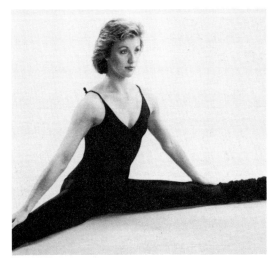

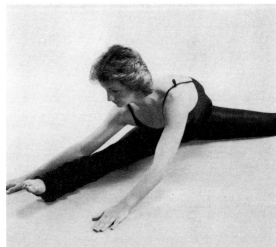

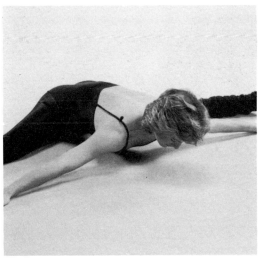

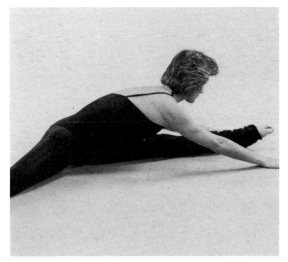

SECOND POSITION FLOOR STRETCH

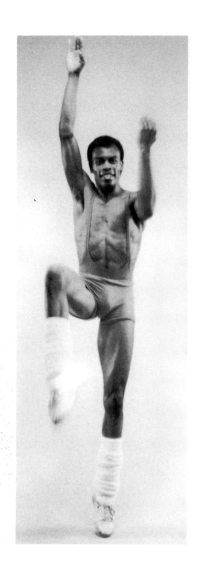

PUTTING IT TOGETHER

The following is a schedule of the aerobics exercises, organized into catagories, beginners, intermediate, and advanced.

If this is the first time that you are doing this type of exercise, regardless of your fitness level, start at the beginners level and progress to intermediate once you have completely mastered the correct form and the exercise routine starts to become easy.

The same principle applies to progressing to the advanced level. When the exercise becomes easy then the intensity must be increased or the benefits will start to diminish, therefore, in progressing to an advanced level the number of exercises increases and the number of repetitions also increases; another way of increasing the intensity is speeding up the pace of performing the movement.

WARM-UP

	Beginner	Intermediate	Advanced
Breathing Arms	8 reps	8 reps	8 reps
Shoulder Lifts	16 reps	24 reps	24 reps
Side Bends	8 sets	12 sets	16 sets
Modern Drop Combo	4 sets	4 sets	4 sets
Waist Isolation	8 sets	16 sets	16 sets
Alternate Ribcage Stretch	8 sets	16 sets	16 sets
Contracted Fly-away	8 reps	16 reps	24 reps
Plie and Stretch	24 reps	24 reps	24 reps
Long Leg Stretch	16 sets	8 sets	8 sets
Roll Up	(transitional movement)		
Contract and Release	8 sets	16 sets	16 sets
Luigi Open Stretch		16 sets	6 sets
4-part Lunge Sequence		6 sets	6 sets

ARMS

	Beginner	Intermediate	Advanced
Shoulder Circles	8 reps	16 reps	16 reps
Hammer Fist	16 reps	24 reps	32 reps
Big Bird	16 reps	24 reps	32 reps
Deltoid Pulse (high) or variation (side)	24 reps	32 reps	64 reps
Deltoid Rotations (front of back)	24 reps	32 reps	64 reps
Scissors	24 reps	32 reps	64 reps
Bicep Curls	16 reps	32 reps	48 reps
Forearm Squeezes	24 reps	32 reps	48 reps
Wrist Curl	24 reps	32 reps	48 reps
Standing Weed Pull	16 reps	32 reps	32 reps
Tricep Extension	16 reps	24 reps	32-48 reps
Tricep Extension Pulse	16 reps	24 reps	32 reps
Tricep Extension Clap	16 reps	24 reps	32 reps
Tricep Rotation	16 reps	24 reps	32 reps

BACK

	Beginner	Intermediate	Advanced
Blade Squeeze Table Top	8 reps	16 reps	24 reps
Big Bird Table Top	16 reps	24 reps	32-48 reps
Second to Elbows	16 reps	24 reps	32-48 reps
Pull Down Isolate	8 reps	16 reps	24-32 reps

CHEST

Peck Deck	16 reps	32 reps	64 reps
Bent Arm Scissors (Cable Squeeze)	16 reps	32 reps	64 reps
Straight Arm Scissors	16 reps	32 reps	64 reps

WAIST

Over Top Stretch	16 sets	24 sets	24 sets
Shoe Lace	8 sets	16 sets	16 sets
Pulling Rope		16 sets	24 sets
Bow and Arrow		16 sets	24 sets
Monkey Pull		16 sets	24 sets
Trunk Twist	8 reps	16 reps	16 reps

PRE-CARDIO

	Beginner	Intermediate	Advanced
Fly-aways	8 reps	16 reps	24 reps
Fly-aways (knees up)		16 reps	24 reps
Toe Touch (with plie)	8 reps	16 reps	24 reps
Toe Touch (with lunge)		16 reps	24 reps
Side-to-Side Toe Touch	8 sets	12 sets	16 sets
Knee Up	8 sets	16 sets	24 sets

CARDIO

Jump Kick Butt	16 reps	32 reps	48 reps
Stride Jumps	24 reps	48 reps	64 reps
Double Knee Up	8 sets	16 sets	24 sets
Running Knee High	16 sets	24 sets	32 sets
Moon Walk	16 sets	24 sets	32 sets
Pendulum (single)	8 sets	16 sets	32 sets
Crosses Small Kicks		24 sets	32 sets
Beats		24 sets	32 sets

LEGS

Side Leg Raise (point)	16 reps	32 reps	64 reps
Side Leg Raise (kick bum)	8 reps	16 reps	24 reps
Side Leg Raise (flex and stretch)	8 reps	16 reps	24 reps
Turn In, Turn Out (flexed foot)	8 reps	16 reps	32 reps
Sitting Chair Legs	8 reps	24 reps	32 reps
Sitting Chair (variation)	8 reps	24 reps	32 reps
Adductor Raise	16 reps	24 reps	32 reps
Adductor Raise (flex and stretch)	8 reps	16 reps	24 reps
Hamstring Tucks	16 reps	32 reps	64 reps

BUTTOCKS

Bum Tucks (variation 1)	16 reps	24 reps	32 reps
Bum Tucks (variation 2)	16 reps	24 reps	32 reps
Bum Tucks (variation 3)	16 reps	24 reps	32 reps
Bum Tucks (variation 5)	16 reps	24 reps	32 reps
Bum Tucks (variation 6)	16 reps	24 reps	32 reps
Doggie Leg (knee lift)	8 reps	24 reps	32 rep
Doggie Leg (variation)		24 reps	24 reps
Doggie Leg Rear Pulse (leg turned out)	16 reps	32 reps	64 reps
Doggie Leg Rear Pulse (flex and stretch)	8 reps	16 reps	16 reps
Doggie Leg Rear Pulse (kick bum)	8 reps	16 reps	16 reps
Doggie Leg Rear Pulse (90-degree angle leg)	8 reps	16 reps	24 reps

ABDOMINALS

Leg Raise 45-90 Degrees (beginners bend knees)	8 reps	24 reps	32 reps
Knee to Chest	8 reps	24 reps	32 reps
Sitting 15-degree Crunch		16 reps	24 reps
Bicycle (hand under bum for beginners)	16 sets	32 sets	64 sets
Bicycle (with extension)			24 sets
Big Walks			24 sets
Crunch (beginners bend knees slightly)	8 reps	24 reps	48 reps
Crunch, feet to ceiling (beginners bend knees)		24 reps	32 reps
Crunch, rub kneecaps	Work until fatigue		
COOL DOWN	Time 3 to 5 Minutes		

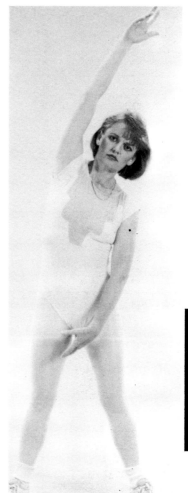

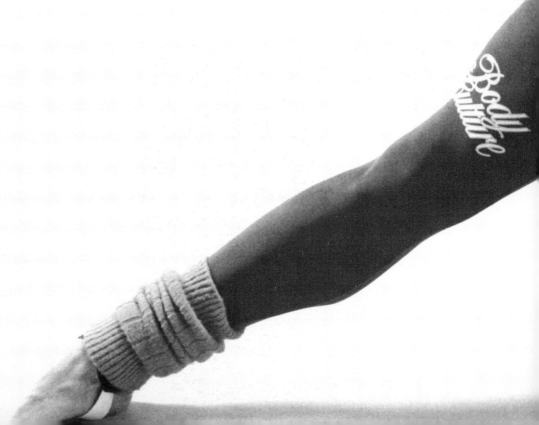

STRETCH

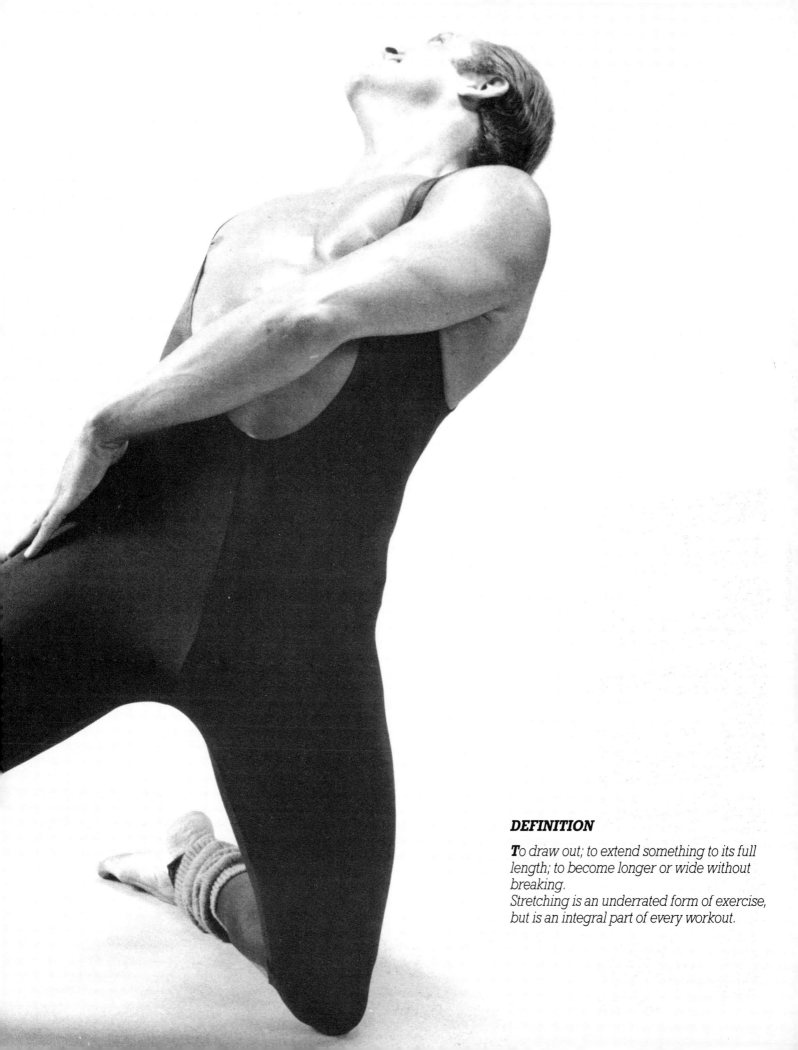

DEFINITION

To draw out; to extend something to its full length; to become longer or wide without breaking.
Stretching is an underrated form of exercise, but is an integral part of every workout.

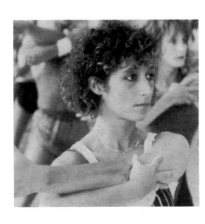

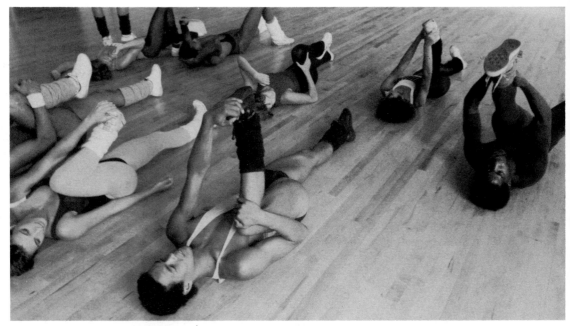

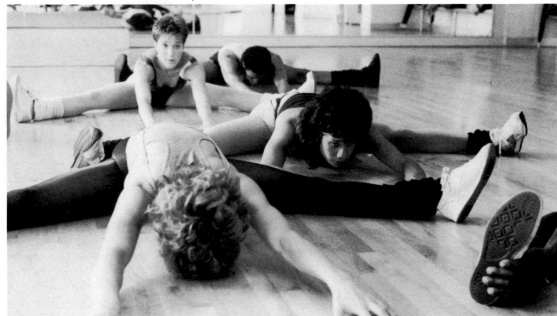

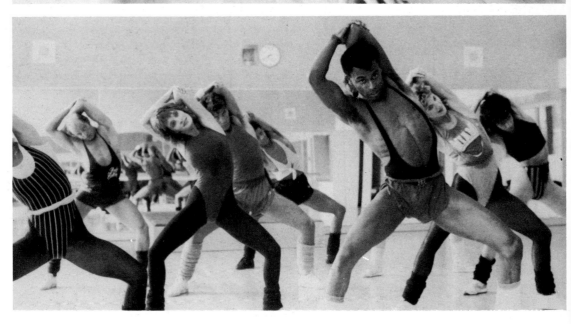

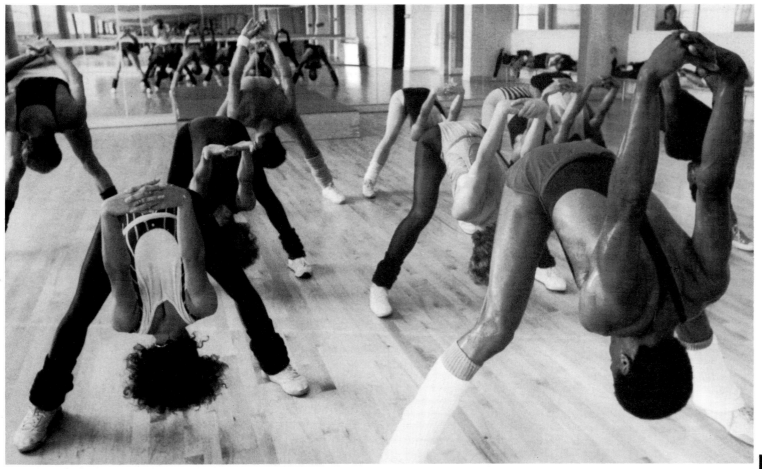

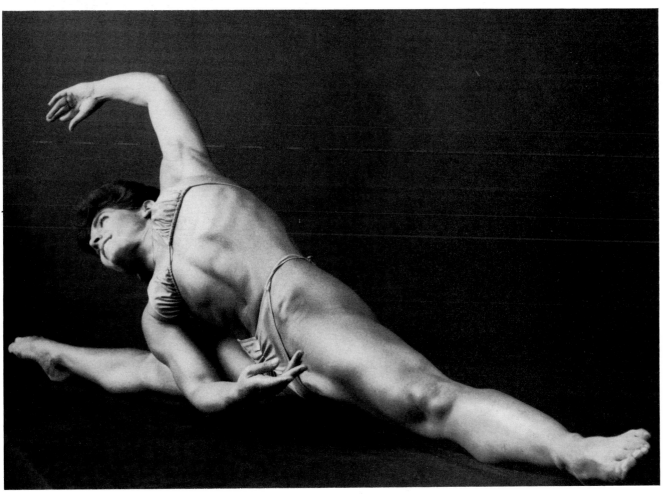

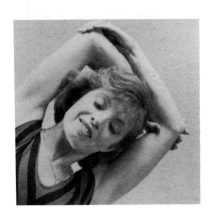

INTRODUCTION AND BENEFITS

It is an undeniable and inescapable fact that, as we age, the body's muscles shorten up. We see examples of this every day when we observe the painfully slow, limited range of movement among many senior citizens. Even among our contemporaries, we may hear complaints about their being unable to do what they were capable of a few years ago.

Regular stretching belongs in everyone's workout regimen. It is the only way to retard this part of the aging process. It has both physical and psychological effects. When you don't move like an oldtimer, you are less apt to look and feel like an oldtimer. Extending the muscles can really help extend the prime of your life!

Since I have been stretching with each workout, my ability to perform the exercises, especially the aerobics classes, has improved. The muscle soreness I used to experience in the 24 to 48 hours following a strenuous workout has lessened greatly and the muscles themselves are less tense, a factor which allows one to flex them harder and achieve better definition.

If you are already very flexible, then stretching exercises are only necessary to maintain that flexibility. Don't take your flexibility for granted – the muscles will shorten without stretching. If you are one of the unfortunate people whose fingers can only come within two feet of the floor when you bend over, then focus your attention on this type of exercise.

BENEFITS OF STRETCHING

- increases flexibility and range of motion.
- reduces soreness experienced after exercise.
- reduces tension in the muscles by helping to eliminate the buildup of toxins.
- increases circulation by stretching and contracting the muscles.
- induces relaxation through slow movements.
- increases body awareness, though focussing on the particular muscles being stretched.
- slows down the natural aging process of shortening muscle fibres.
- enhances athletic performance by improving your coordination via an easier and increased range of motion.
- reduces the possibility of injury; when a muscles is stretched before an exercise, it can better withstand the stress imposed on it.

METHODS OF STRETCHING

The old method of stretching which many young people learned on football fields, in gymnastics and in the military service involved bouncing up and down in a bent-over position to touch the toes. The upper body's weight was used to force a stretch of the hamstrings.

This is known as ballistic stretching. In many cases, it has been found to be ineffective because of a protective body mechanism known as the stretch reflex. When the nerve endings in the muscle sense that the muscle is being stretched too far, they send out a signal for the muscle to contract, to prevent the muscle from overstretching and damaging the tissues.

Overstretching or use of the ballistic method can actually lead to a muscle-tear type of injury because you are much less aware of the stretch limitations of the muscle. You must govern the stretch, not gravity.

Slow controlled stretching is the method of choice. Assume the proper form and alignment as described in the text to ease into the stretch. Beginners go just to the point of slight discomfort, back off a little, then hold the pose for the recommended time. You will feel the muscle relaxing. The tension actually releases. This is the goal of your initial stretching program.

Each person has his own degree of flexibility and there is no advantage in competing with others in this aspect of exercise. Stretching is a personal, relaxing type of exercise, not aggressive and competitive. Some of your joints will be more flexible than others. This is common and not a cause for concern.

IMPROVING YOUR STRETCH

Once you are accustomed to the initial stretching method, gradually try to increase your degree of stretch. As you feel the muscular tension release, increase the stretch to a point of mild discomfort and back off slightly. Keep edging it further as it releases. Never go too far, or too fast. If it hurts, you have gone too far and must ease off immediately. In stretching, pain means that you are causing some damage.

BREATHING

Slow, rhythmic, accentuated breathing is a technique that facilitates improved stretching. Visualize more oxygen getting to the muscles being stretched. This adds greatly to the degree of relaxation achieved.

OVERSTRETCHING

A muscle may be overstretched in different ways. We have already mentioned how a ballistic-type stretch can cause a reflex contraction in a muscle. Bouncing too hard at this point can tear the muscle, or worse, the ligaments.

In the slow controlled stretch, there is a risk of exaggerating the stretch into the area of extreme discomfort and pain. This is not advised, as it can result in injuries.

Holding a stretch for too long a period of time can also overstretch the muscles. Don't try to set a record. Listen to your body. It will tell you when you have stretched long enough.

There is also a risk of concentrating too much on stretching one muscle or group of muscles. This is common in many stretch classes where instructors over-emphasize the hamstring, as though it were the only muscle that needs to be stretched.

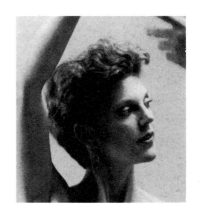

Stretching should not leave the muscles sore. When done properly, its purpose is to relieve muscle soreness. If the muscle is sore after stretching, chances are that you have overstretched. The exception to this, of course, is the rank beginner, who has done no form of exercise for a period of years. For these people, stretching itself may be strenuous exercise and they will have to endure some soreness.

WARM-UP

Some people use stretching as a method of warming up for other exercises. Be warned that you cannot properly stretch a cold muscle. Stretches should be preceded by some mild form of exercise, such as a general loosening up – walking, shaking the arms, twisting, mild aerobics or doing the actual stretch positions, but not holding the stretch.

In my routine at the gym, I begin with five minutes on an exercise bike at low tension to loosen up and get the blood circulating to the muscles. I follow this with sit-ups for 12 to 15 minutes. Only then do I perform my stretches – after the warm-up and before the actual workout.

Stretching is also an excellent cool-down at the end of the workout. It helps to slow down the pace and will help to prevent muscle soreness from intensive workouts.

Stretching must be included in everyone's routine, no matter what the level. As you get older, it becomes even more important.

STRETCH

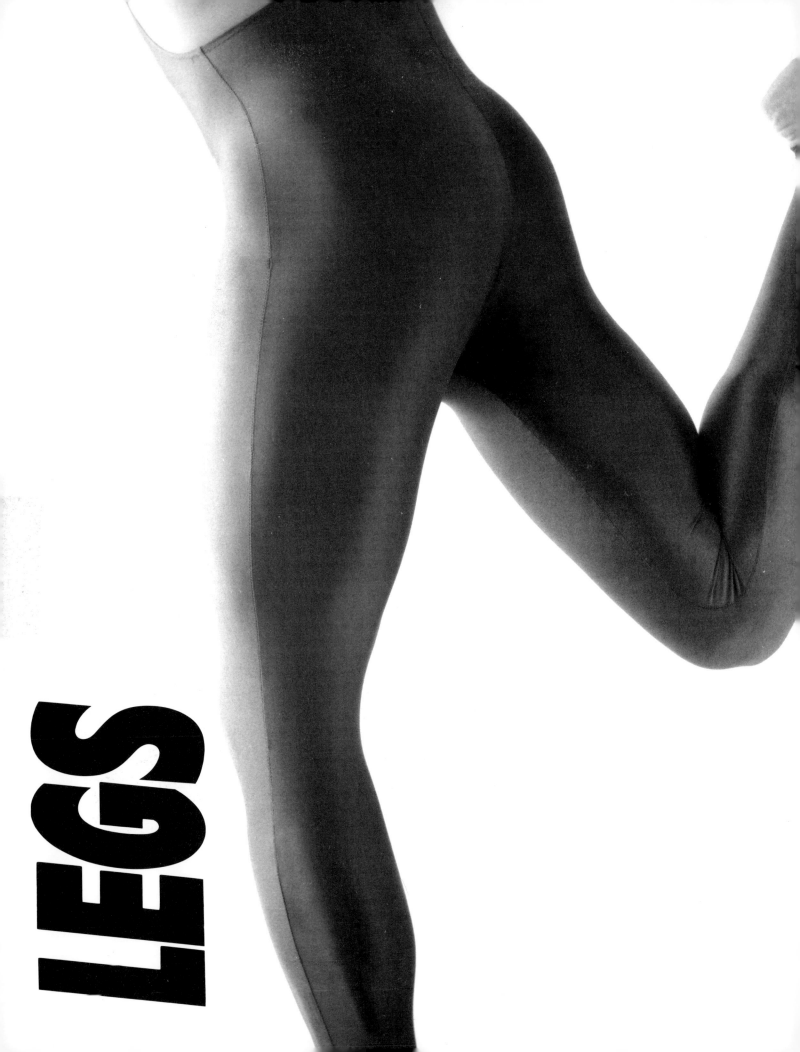

LEGS

LEG STRETCHES

STANDING QUAD

Emphasis:
Upper middle quadriceps.

Position:
Stand, holding something for balance, if desired. Bend the left knee and bring the heel toward the buttocks. Grasp that ankle with the left hand and bring the ankle as close as possible to the buttocks.

Form:
Lift the ankle by pushing the knee back and lifting the ankle with the hand, keeping the heel as close as possible to the buttocks. Hold for 15 seconds, then repeat for other side.

LYING QUAD

Emphasis:
Quadriceps.

Position:
Lie on your right side. Supporting your head with the right hand, bend the left knee and grasp the top of the foot with the left hand. The right leg is positioned slightly forward for balance.

Form:
Lift the heel by pushing the knee back and pulling the foot with the hand. The foot is pulled back and away from the body.

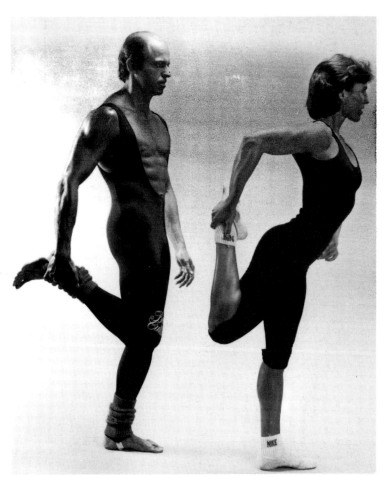

STANDING QUAD

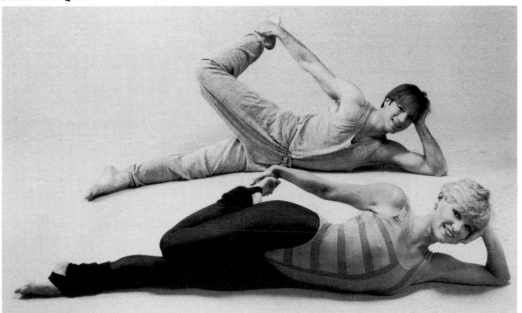

LYING QUAD

141

KNEELING QUAD (single)

Emphasis:
Upper quadriceps.

Position:
Kneel on both knees. Slide the left knee back as far as possible and grab the left ankle with the left hand. Place the right hand on the floor, to the inside of the knee, to support and balance the upper body.

Form:
Pull the left ankle forward. Slide the knee back and hold the stretch.

KNEELING QUAD (both)

Emphasis:
Quadriceps and front of ankles.

Position:
Kneel on a carpet or pad. The feet are positioned just outside the buttocks, with the line of the foot and the line of the thigh in the same direction.

Form:
Lean back, using both arms for support. Go back as far as possible and hold the stretch. Women can generally go further than men in this stretch.

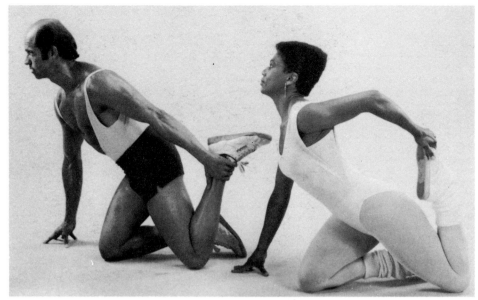

KNEELING QUAD (single)

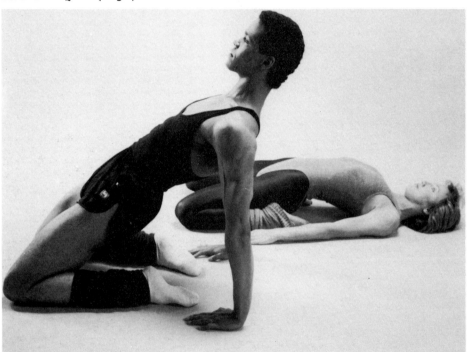

KNEELING QUAD (both)

HAMSTRING STRETCHES

STANDING HAMSTRING

Emphasis:
Hamstrings, top and bottom, with some emphasis on the upper calf.

Position:
Stand, with feet together, and bend over, sliding the hands down the outsides of the legs.

Form:
Grab the ankles and slowly pull the head toward the knees.
Variations may be done with the feet apart. Feet shoulder width apart stresses the upper medial hamstring; a wider stance stresses the lower middle hamstring. The exercise may also be done sitting, with one leg straight, the other slightly bent, for isolation.

HURDLE STRETCH

Emphasis:
Quadriceps.

Position:
Sit with one leg stretched straight in front and the other bent back at 45 to 90 degrees. Lean back, sliding the supporting hand out, to lower the back toward the floor. The bent knee will come up slightly.

Form:
Slowly, press the knee back down as close as possible to the floor.

CAUTION! If this proves hard on your knees or if you have had previous knee damage, such as a cartilage or ligament tear, stick with the other quad stretches. It is not advisable to do this stretch until the knee is fully healed. Even then, approach with caution.

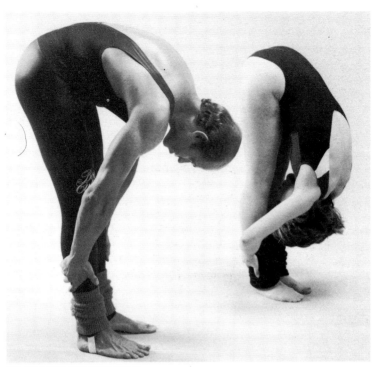

STANDING HAMSTRING

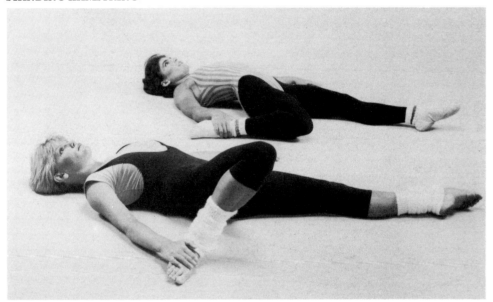

HURDLE STRETCH

143

KNEE TO CHEST

Emphasis:
Hamstrings and middle gluteals.

Position:
Lie supine and bring the knee to your chest.

Form:
Clasp the hands over the knee and pull it closer to the chest. Keep the hands and lower back flat. Hold the stretch and repeat for the opposite side.

A variation may be performed from the bent-leg position. Keeping the knee to the chest, grab back of the ankle or calf and slowly extend the leg as far as possible. The more flexible you are, the closer the hand will be to the ankle. The opposite leg may bend a little on this one. This variation empasizes the lower and middle hamstring.

SITTING SECOND POSITION

Emphasis:
Middle and lower hamstring.

Position:
Sit with your legs in second position. Turn the upper body toward one leg and bend forward. Grab that leg at the calf or the ankle, depending on your flexibility. Keep the opposite hip on the floor.

Form:
Pull the middle chest toward the thigh and keep that foot flexed.

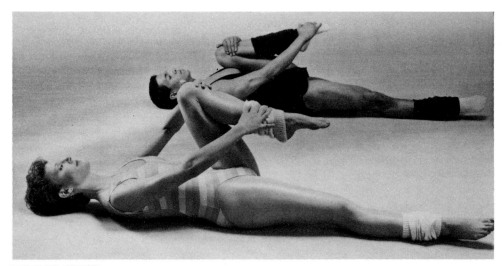

KNEE TO CHEST

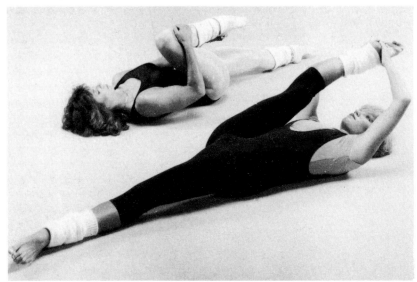

VARIATION

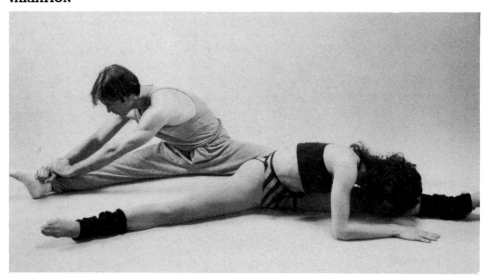

SITTING SECOND POSITION

144

BAR

Emphasis:
Middle lower hamstring.

Position:
Facing the bar or the table, place one foot upon it and flex the foot. Grab the ankle.

Form:
Pull the middle chest toward the thigh and hold as close as possible. For a variation, you may change the height of the bar.

SITTING ONE LEG

Emphasis:
Middle lower hamstring.

Position:
Sit with both legs straight out in front. Bend the right knee and grab the ankle or calf.

Form:
Keeping the thigh as close as possible to the chest, fully extend the knee, slowly pushing the heel toward the ceiling.
A variation may be performed this way: sit with the left leg bent and resting on the floor. Bend the right knee and bring it close to the chest. Grasp the ankle and straighten the leg up, pressing the heel toward the ceiling.

LYING SUPINE

Emphasis:
Upper hamstring and buttocks.

Position:
Lie with one leg straight on the floor and the other bent toward the chest. Bring the knee to the opposite shoulder and roll the hip, so that the pelvic line is perpendicular to the floor. Grab the ankle or calf with the opposite hand.

Form:
Slowly extend this leg, with the foot flexed. Keep the knee and hip in the same position, as high as possible.

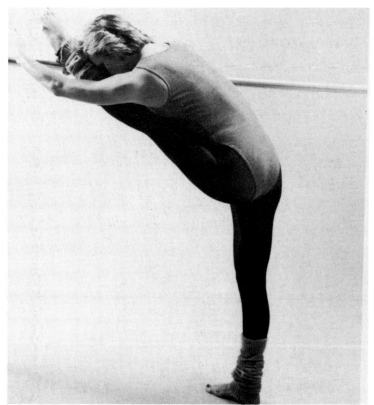

BAR

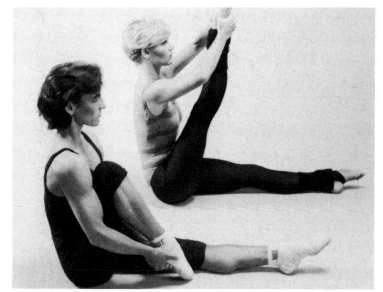

SITTING ONE LEG

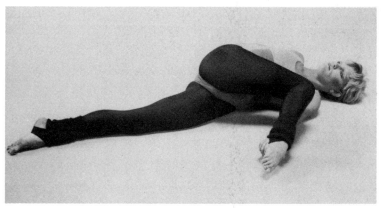
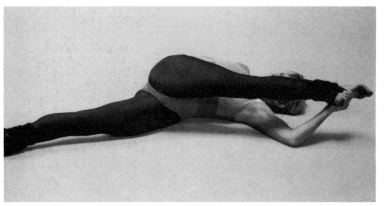

LYING SUPINE

CALF STRETCHES

BENT OVER, HANDS ON FLOOR

Emphasis:
Lower calf.

Position:
Kneel on all fours, with the feet together. Straighten the legs and raise the lower body up on the toes. Keep the feet together and hands on the floor.

Form:
After your are up on your toes, begin to press the heel down toward the floor and hold the stretch.
Do a variation by stretching one calf at a time for variation. You may also decrease the angle of the upper body, by moving the hands closer to the feet. As the angle is decreased, the emphasis of the stretch moves higher on the calf.

TOES AGAINST WALL

Emphasis:
Middle and upper calf.

Position:
Fully flex one foot. Place the toe against the wall and fully extend the knee. Keep the other foot back six to eight inches for balance.

Form:
Keep the body and the leg straight and lean forward. Changing the foot position will alter the stress – turning the foot in stresses the medial calf; turning the foot out stresses the lateral calf.

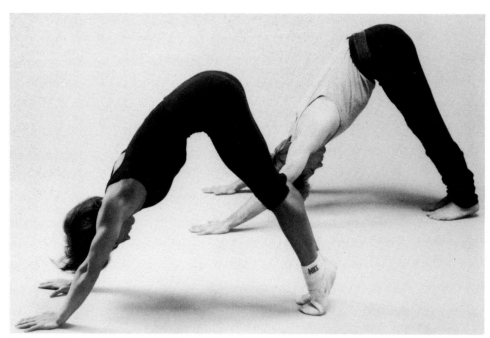

BENT OVER, HANDS ON FLOOR

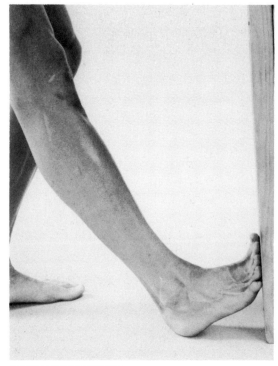 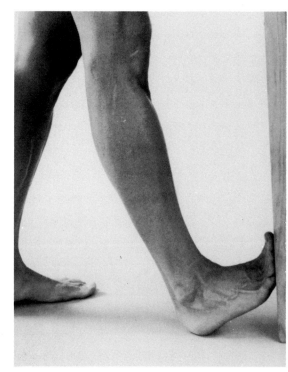

TOES AGAINST WALL

TOES ELEVATED

Emphasis:
Middle calf.

Position:
Stand on the edge of a block, holding something for balance.

Form:
Slowly lower the heels as far as possible and hold the stretch. You may do singles, isolating one leg at a time, or use foot positions that are turned in or turned out to alter the stretch.

SITTING PULL

Emphasis:
Calf.

Position:
Sit with the legs together in front of you and bend the right knee. Grab the ball of that foot with both hands and flex the foot.

Form:
Slowly straighten the leg and pull the ball of the foot toward you. Hold the stretch.
This exercise may be done with both legs at the same time or as an assisted stretch, in which a training partner applies the pressure and raises your heel off the floor one to two inches.

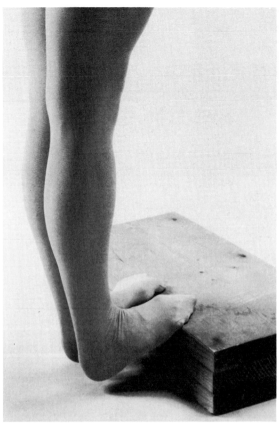 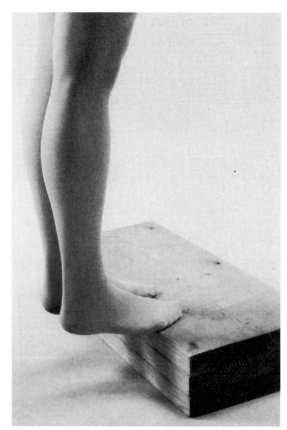

TOES ELEVATED

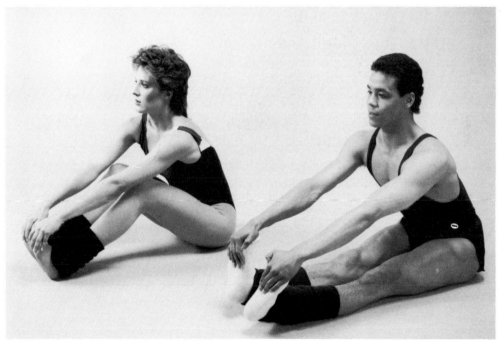

SITTING PULL

BACK

BACK STRETCHES

SITTING POSITION (1)

Emphasis:
Middle and lower back.

Position:
Sit with the feet about 12 inches apart in front of you and the knees slightly bent.

Form:
Round your back, bring the chin forward toward the chest and bend forward. The hands slide down the outside of the legs to grab the ankles or calf. Slowly try to pull yourself down toward the floor. If the hamstrings feel stretched, bend the knees a little more to avoid this.

SITTING POSITION (2)

Emphasis:
Lower erector spinae and latissimus dorsi, isolating one side at a time.

Position:
Start as in the previous exercise, but grab the outside of the right foot with your left hand. Keep your arm straight. Twist the body toward the right side. Place the right hand on the floor, beside the buttocks.

Form:
Reach further with the outstretched hand and twist slightly. Hold for 15 seconds and repeat on the other side. Both of these sitting position exercises may be done standing.

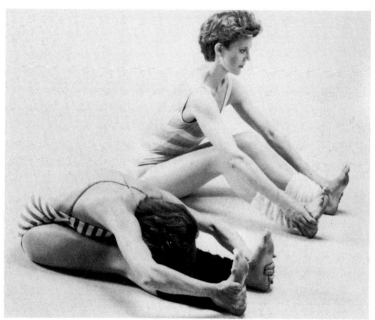

SITTING POSITION (1)

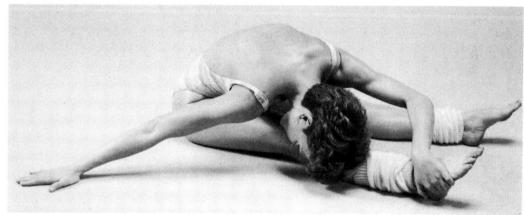

SITTING POSITION (2)

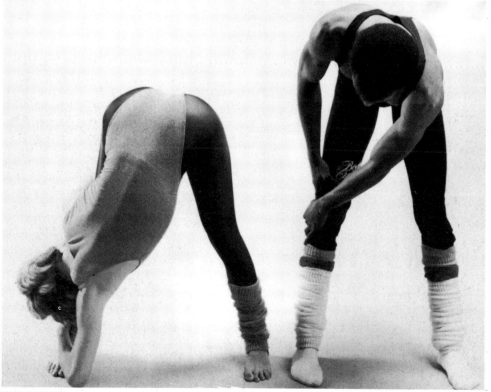

VARIATION

149

LAT STRETCH

Emphasis:
Full latissimus, unilaterally.

Position:
You will need a support structure for resistance in this stretch, a door knob, door jamb, a bar or training partner. Stand facing your support, about 12 inches away. Place your feet shoulder width apart, with the left foot in front of the right. Bend over at 90 degrees and grab the support structure with your right hand.

Form:
Lean away from the support and twist the right hip away from the support. Hold for 15 seconds, then repeat for the other side.

OVERHEAD ELBOW CLASP

Emphasis:
Upper latissimus. The lower latissimus is stressed a little more with the twisting action.

Position:
Lift the left arm over the head and flex the forearm at 90 degrees. Grab the left elbow with the right hand. Be careful to keep the bent arm in this position. If you pull it too much beyond 90 degrees, it becomes a tricep stretch.

Form:
Lift the left shoulder. Elongate the left side of the ribcage. Bend to the right slightly and pull downward with the right hand. For added stretch, twist toward the right. Repeat for the opposite side.

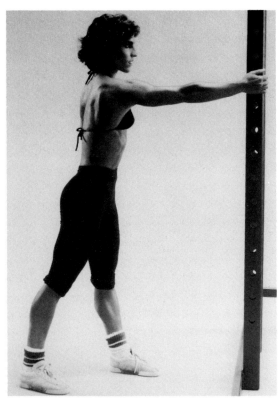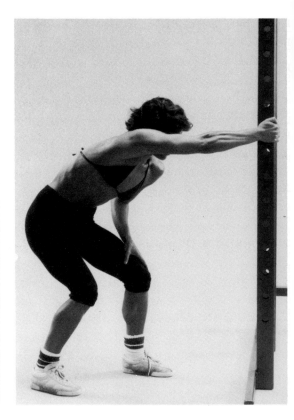

LAT STRETCH

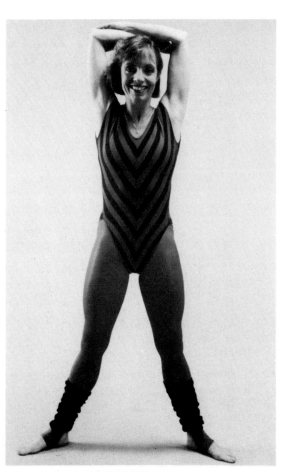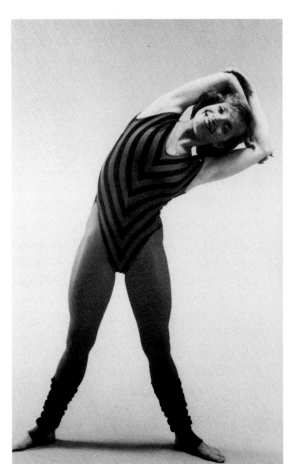

OVERHEAD ELBOW CLASP

FRONT SHOULDER CRAB

Emphasis:
Trapezius and rhomboids.

Position:
Stand erect and cross your arms to place the hands on opposite shoulders. Keep the elbows up at shoulder height. Round the upper back.

Form:
Bend forward from the waist slightly, pulling the shoulders forward and rounding the upper back even more.

ASSISTED NECK FLEXION

Emphasis:
Neck and upper middle back.

Position:
Stand with your feet apart and clasp your hands behind your head.

Form:
Pull the head and upper spine forward with very light pressure from the hands. Bring the chin to the chest, then flex further if you can, to extend the stretch to the upper middle back. Hold for 15 seconds.

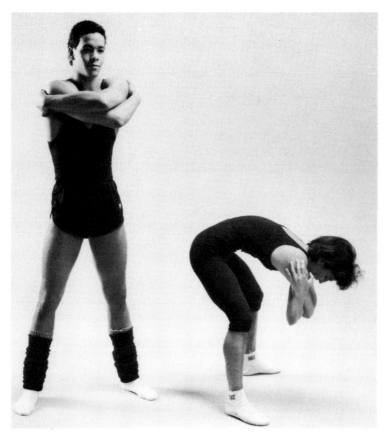

FRONT SHOULDER CRAB

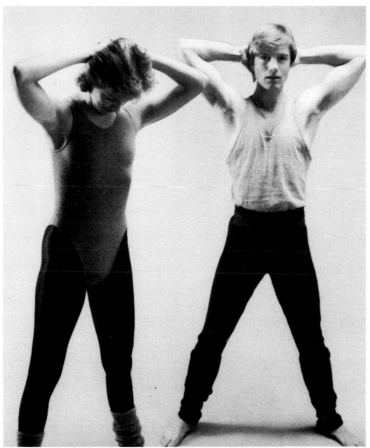

ASSISTED NECK FLEXION

CHEST

DOOR STRETCH

Emphasis:
Upper and outer chest and deltoids.

Position:
Stand in a doorway and grasp the sides of the door with the arms down at about 30 degrees. (We have used a power rack instead of a doorway in our example.) Hold your chin up.

Form:
Lean forward, arching the back and keeping chin up and the shoulders down.

PECK DECK POSITION

Emphasis:
Middle and lower chest if the feet are in the doorway; upper and outer chest if the feet are back from the doorway.

Position:
Stand with the arms up, the upper arms parallel to the floor and the forearms resting on the door jamb. Keep the chin up. the feet may be directly in the doorway or back 18 to 24 inches.

Form:
Lean forward through the doorway, stretching forward with the chin. This stresses the muscles in the upper middle chest.

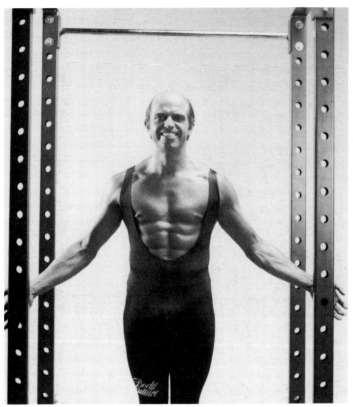
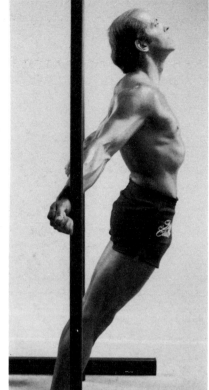

DOOR STRETCH

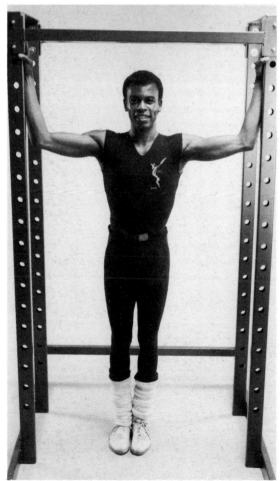
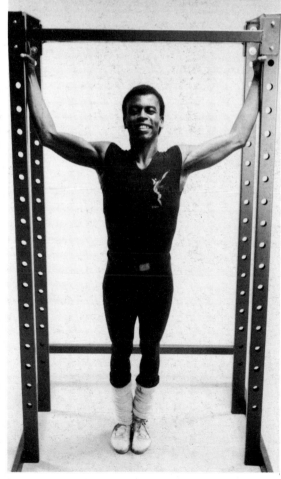

PECK DECK POSITION

ONE ARM AT A TIME

Emphasis:
Upper and outer chest.

Position 1:
Step through the doorway, then reach back with the right hand and grab the door jamb at shoulder height. Put the right foot across in front of the left, a full stride.

Form:
Lift and rotate the right side of the chest, while twisting the torso to the left and leaning in that direction.

Position 2:
You may vary this by placing the left hand at the top of the door jamb. The feet are positioned in the doorway at a 45-degree angle and the upper body is parallel to the door. Lean forward and rotate toward the right side. this stresses the full outside chest.

HANDS BEHIND HEAD

Emphasis:
Upper middle chest.

Position:
Stand and clasp the hands behind the head, chin out, elbows back.

Form:
Raise the chest up and press the elbows back as far as possible. Hold the stretch.
For a variation, have the hands out to the side at 45 degrees, then press back and lift the chest up and out.

HANDS BEHIND BACK

Emphasis:
Middle and outer chest.

Position:
Stand with the hands interlocked behind the back, palms up. Stretch the hands down and back, the chin up and out.

Form:
Pull the arms back as far as possible and push the chin out and up as far as possible.

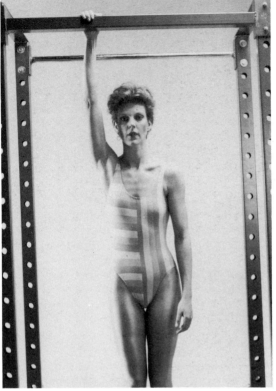

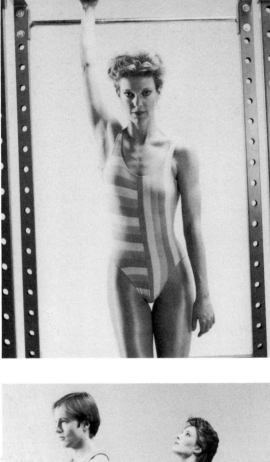

ONE ARM AT AT TIME

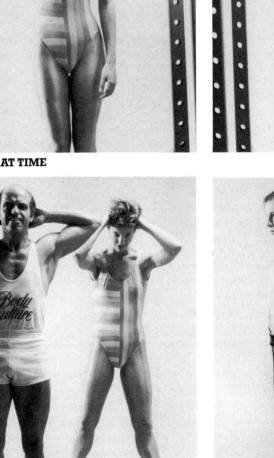

HANDS BEHIND HEAD

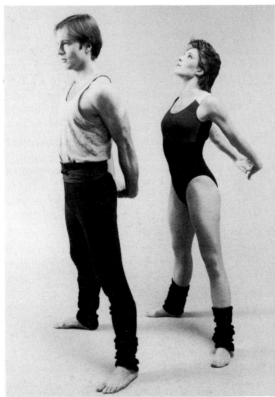

HANDS BEHIND BACK

LYING ON STOMACH

Emphasis:
Upper and outer chest.

Position:
Lie face down, with the left arm outstretched at 90 degrees. The right hand is in the push-up position by the right shoulder.

Form:
Keep the left shoulder close to the floor. Push up and rotate the right side of the upper body to the left side. Reach out with the left arm at the same time.

SITTING

Emphasis:
Middle and outer chest, with some work on the shoulder and bicep. If the stretch is done with hands at shoulder width, there is more emphasis on the middle chest.

Position:
Sit with the legs out straight, hands on the floor behind the body and spaced six to eight inches wider than shoulder width.

Form:
Slide the hands out a little and raise the chest and chin up and out as far as possible.

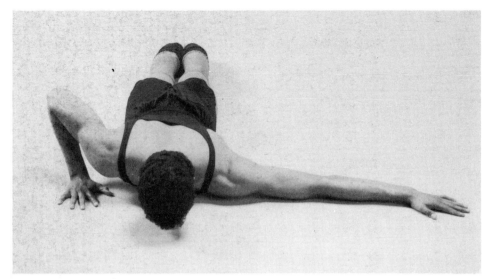

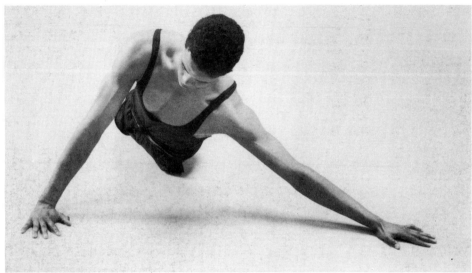

LYING ON STOMACH

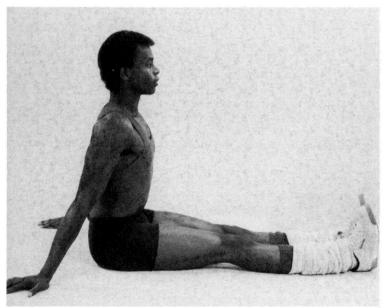

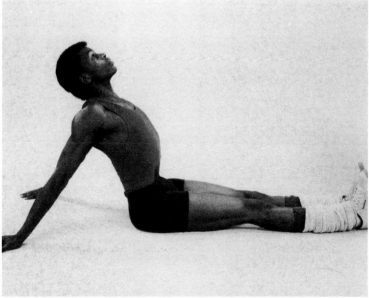

SITTING

155

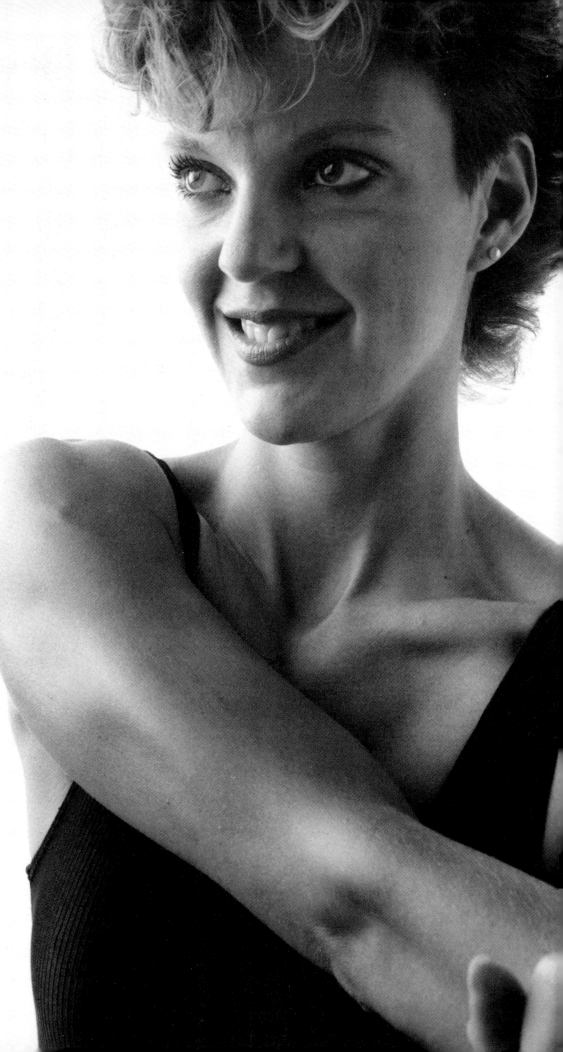

SHOULDERS

SHOULDER STRETCHES

DOORWAY STRETCH, UPPER POSITION

Emphasis:
Rear deltoid (underarm), latissimus, ribcage and pectorals.

Position:
Stand in a doorway with your hands directly overhead, holding on to the top of the frame.

Form:
Lean forward, arching the stomach out, and come up on the toes. Keep the arms straight. At the same time, lean to accentuate the stretch and hold it for 15 to 20 seconds.

Variations:
Take a deep breath, hold it, then lean further through the doorway. This also stretches the lower ribs and arms. A wide grip will affect the rear deltoid and lats. If you are tall, you may need to lean further through the doorway or bend the knees.

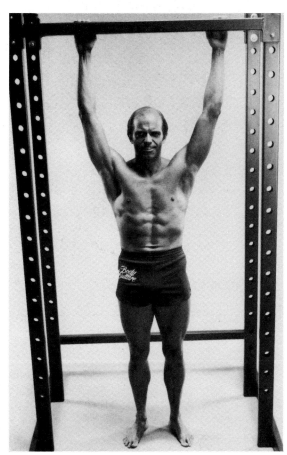

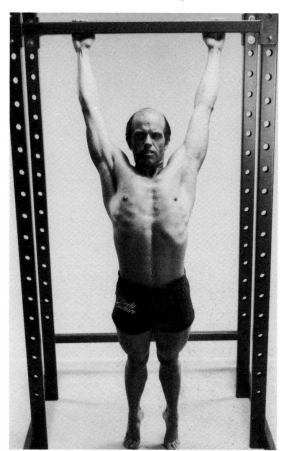

DOORWAY STRETCH

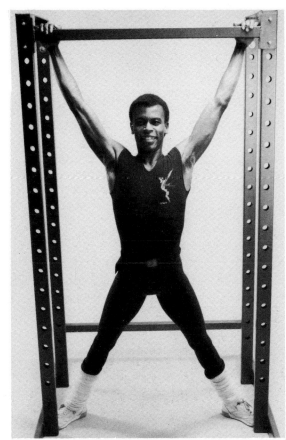

VARIATION

STRETCH

ONE-ARM DOORWAY

Emphasis:
Pectorals, latissimus, rear deltoids (underarm) and ribcage.

Position:
Stand in a doorway and raise one arm directly above to grasp the top of the door frame.

Form:
Lean forward, arching the stomach out, and rise up on your toes. Keep the arms straight and hold for 15 to 20 seconds.
To emphasize the rear deltoid, do the stretch with a twist to the side opposite the raised arm.

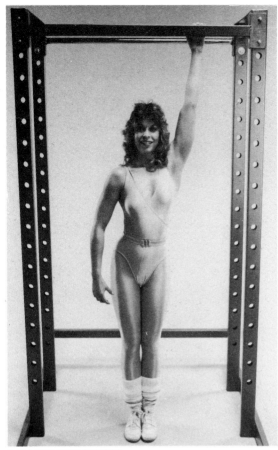 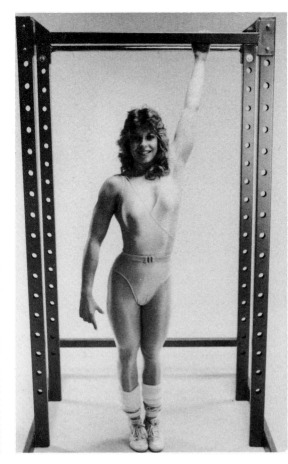

ONE-ARM DOORWAY

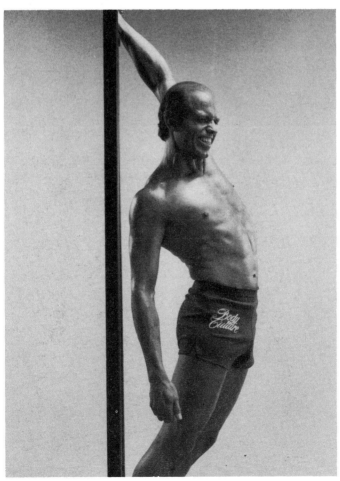

VARIATION

158

ONE ARM CROSS STRETCH, DOORWAY

Emphasis:
Deltoids.

Position:
Stand with one foot inside the doorway, facing the door jamb. With the arm furthest from the door, reach across and grab the other side of the door jamb at shoulder height.

Form:
Twist the upper body toward the crossed arm. The free hand may also be placed higher on the door frame to aid in pulling the body toward the crossed arm.
Varying the height of the crossed arm shifts the emphasis. At shoulder height, it works the middle deltoid. Six to eight inches above shoulder height works the rear deltoid.

ONE ARM CROSS STRETCH

Emphasis:
Rear and middle deltoids.

Position:
Put your arms in front of you and grab the right elbow with the left hand.

Form:
Pull the right elbow across the chest at shoulder height, toward the left shoulder. Hold for 15 seconds, then repeat for opposite side.

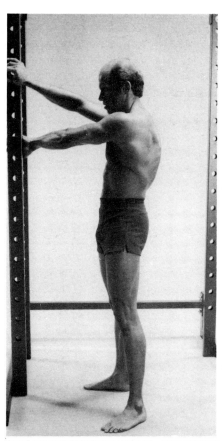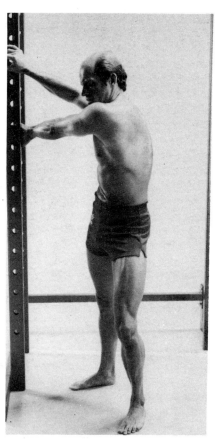

ONE ARM CROSS STRETCH, DOORWAY

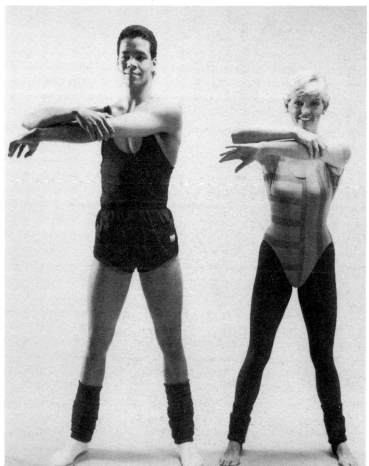

ONE ARM CROSS STRETCH

STRETCH

159

PARTNER SHOULDER STRETCH

Emphasis:
Middle deltoids.

Position:
Stand beside your partner, facing opposite directions, so that the outsides of your left feet are together. Reach over and grasp each other's right hand. The assisting partner reaches under the right hands and grasps your left elbow with his left hand, thumb down. You keep your shoulders square and level.

Form:
The assisting partner pulls your right arm across your chest, while stabilizing you with his left hand. Change roles to stretch your partner's shoulder. To stretch left shoulders, move to the opposite side, right feet together.

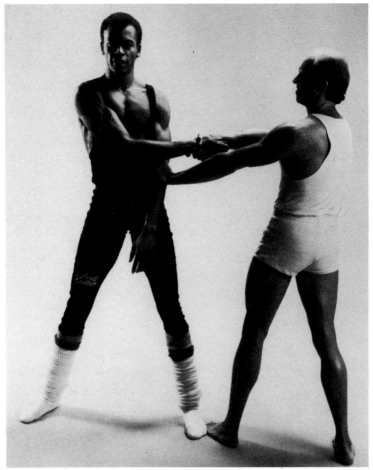

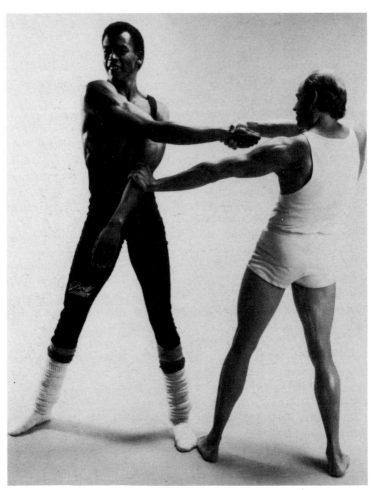

160

BEND OVER A POSITION

Emphasis:
Front and middle deltoids.

Position:
Place feet shoulder width apart and bend the knees slightly. Interlock your fingers behind your buttocks. Stretch the hands down and back and bend forward to 90 degrees or more.

Form:
Raise the arms up as high as possible and hold the stretch for 15 seconds.

DOOR KNOB

Emphasis:
Front and middle deltoids.

Position:
With your back at the edge of the door, reach behind you and grab the doorknob with both hands. Your feet should be about 12 inches away from the door.

Form:
Bend the knees slowly, until you feel a good stretch though the shoulders. Hold for 15 seconds.
This can also be done with an assisting partner holding your wrists behind you and extending the arms backward before the knees are bent.

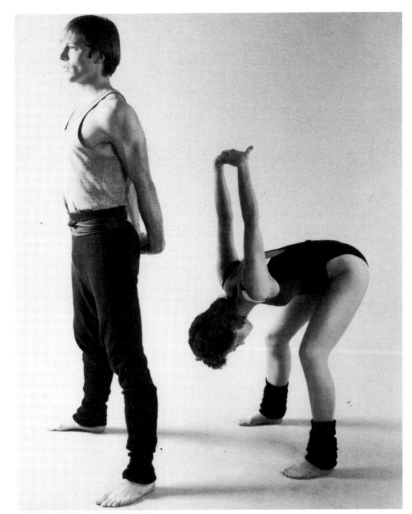

BEND OVER A POSITION

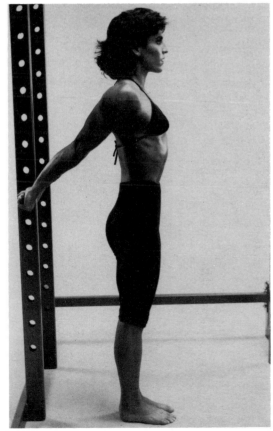

DOOR KNOB

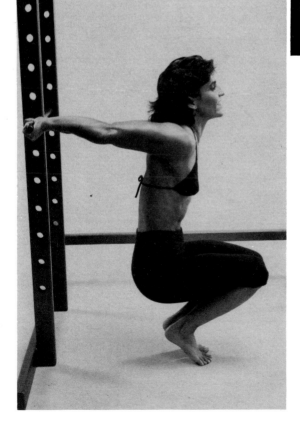

STRETCH

161

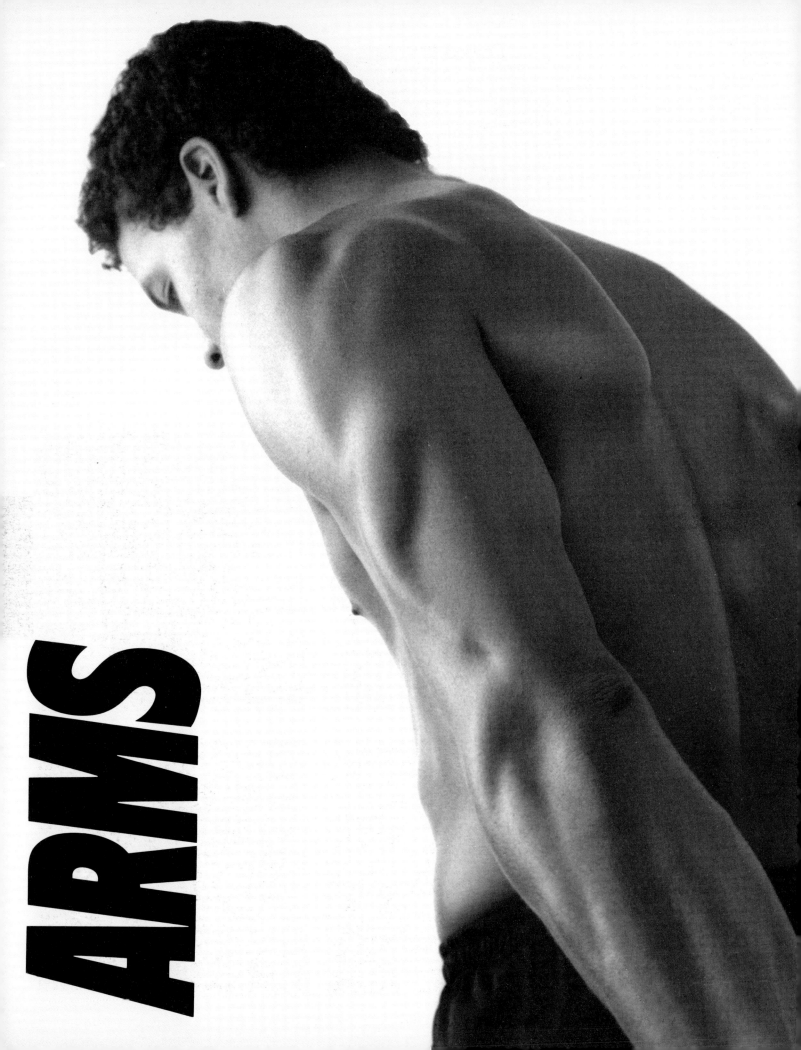

ARMS

ARMS

TRICEP STRETCH

Emphasis:
Triceps.

Position:
Raise the right arm up alongside the head, then flex the arm at the elbow as much as possible, putting the hand behind the head or further. Grasp the right elbow with the left hand.

Form:
Pull the elbow straight across the back toward the left side and hold the stretch. Repeat for opposite side.

WALL STRETCH

Emphasis:
Inside head of triceps.

Position:
Stand facing the wall, 12 to 18 inches away. Raise one arm up and flex the elbow. Place the elbow on the wall and slide it up high.

Form:
Lean in towards the wall. Keep the body straight, the shoulders square to the wall and hold the stretch. Repeat for the opposite side.

ASSISTED TRICEP STRETCH

Emphasis:
Inner and outer head of tricep.

Position:
Stand in fourth position, raise the left arm and flex at the elbow, placing your hand behind your head. Your partner stands to the side of the raised arm. He grabs your left wrist with one hand and your left elbow with his other hand.

Form:
The assisting partner gently pulls down on the left wrist, simultaneously lifting your left elbow up and back. Hold the stretch for 15 seconds, then repeat for the opposite side.
The focus of the stretch is on the inner head of the tricep if the pull is straight back; on the outer head if the pull is more behind the neck.

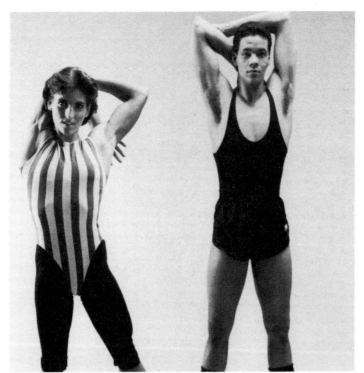

TRICEP STRETCH

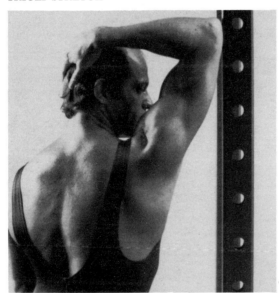

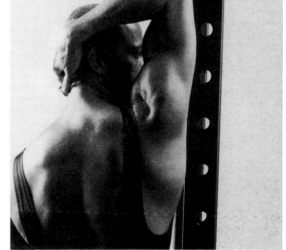

WALL STRETCH

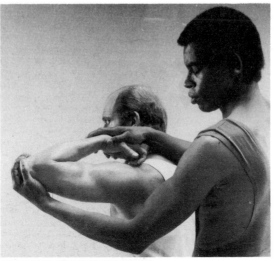

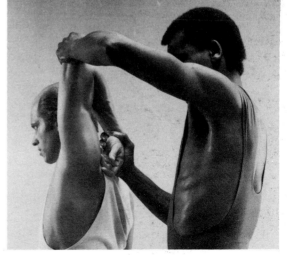

ASSISTED TRICEP STRETCH

BICEPS

ASSISTED FRONT LEAN

Emphasis:
Biceps.

Position:
Stand with your feet shoulder width apart, and your arms about 45 degrees out from your sides, the palms facing forward. Your partner stands behind you and grabs your wrists.

Form:
Your partner balances you and pulls your arms up and slightly together as you lean forward. Hold the stretch for 15 seconds.

BICEP STRETCH

Emphasis:
Biceps, with slight stress on front deltoids.

Position:
Stand in second position, with arms at your sides, palms forward. Extend the wrists fully, until the palms face the floor.

Form:
Pull the arms back as far as you can and hold the stretch for 15 seconds.

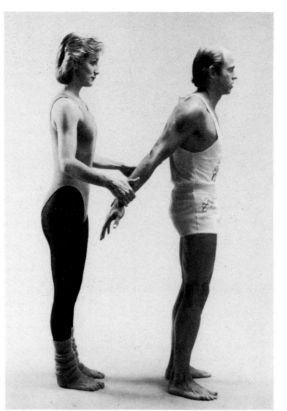 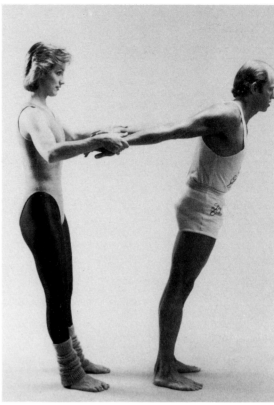

ASSISTED FRONT LEAN

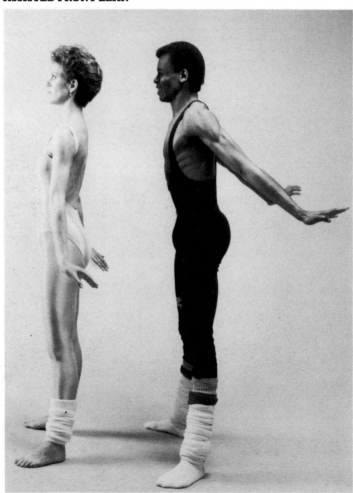

BICEP STRETCH

WRISTS AND FOREARMS

ALL FOUR STRETCH, FLEXORS

Emphasis:
Forearm flexors and wrists.

Position:
Kneel on all fours, with palms on the floor. Turn your hands completely inward, so the fingers are toward you and the thumbs out.

Form:
Keep the palms flat on the floor and lean back. Hold the stretch for 15 seconds.

ALL FOUR STRETCH, EXTENSORS

Emphasis:
Forearm extensors and wrists.

Position:
Kneel on all fours with the palms of the hand up and fingers toward you.

Form:
Lean back, keeping the front of your hands on the floor.

ASSISTED WRIST STRETCH

Emphasis:
Front aspect of wrist.

Position:
Put the left wrist in hyperflexion, by bending the left hand back, and placing the right palm on top of it.

Form:
The right hand gently assists the wrist stretch by exaggerating the flexion. Repeat for the opposite side.
The natural variation for this is assisted wrist hyperextension. Bend the hand forward, then use the opposite hand to gently exaggerate this stretch.

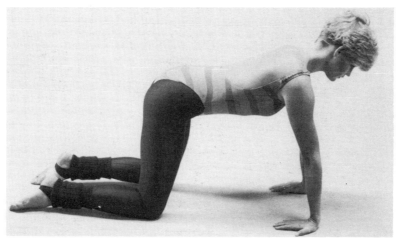

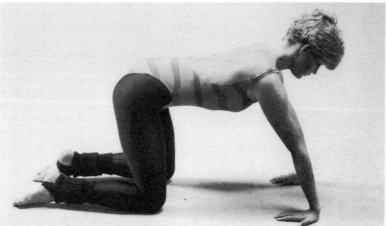

ALL FOUR STRETCH, FLEXORS

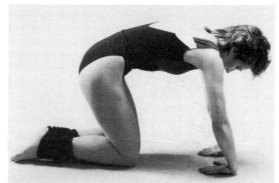

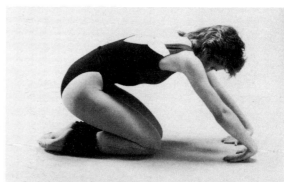

ALL FOUR STRETCH, EXTENSORS

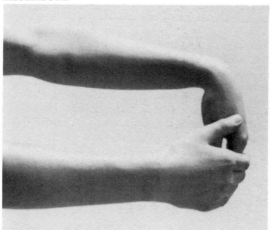

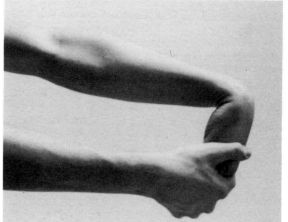

ASSISTED WRIST STRETCH

BUTTOCK

HIPS AND BUTTOCKS

LYING KNEE TO CHEST

Emphasis:
Middle hamstring and outer buttocks.

Position:
Lie on your back and bring the right knee to your chest. Keeping the pelvis and lower back on the floor, grab the right knee with the right hand and the top of the foot with the left hand. Pull the right foot toward the left.

Form:
Pull the knee straight in to the chest. Keep the other leg straight.
You can vary this by pulling the knee toward the opposite shoulder. This emphasizes the outer gluteal piraformus and sacroilliac joints.

GRAM STRETCH

Emphasis:
Gluteus maximus.

Position:
Sit with your left leg extended and the right knee flexed. Place the right heel on the outside of the left knee. Now, bring the left hand over the right knee.

Form:
Pull the right knee towards the left shoulder. Try to keep the left buttock on the floor. Hold the stretch for 15 seconds, then repeat for opposite side.
Advanced trainees may have to reach through with the arms and pull the knee with the elbow. Very flexible individuals may flex the extended leg to just beside the buttocks. Perform the stretch in the same manner.

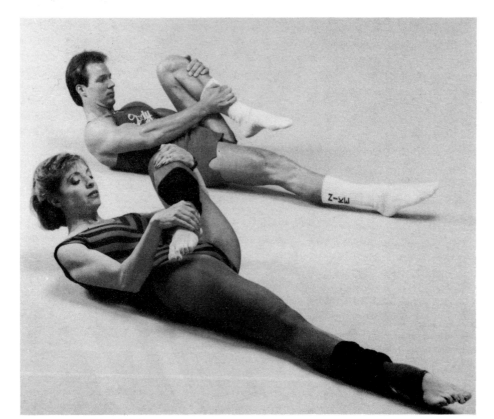

LYING KNEE TO CHEST

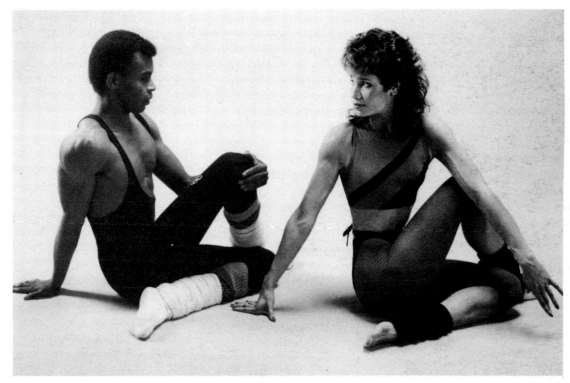

GRAM STRETCH

FOURTH POSITION GLUTEAL STRETCH

Emphasis:
Gluteus maximus and outer gluteals.

Position:
Lie supine, with your left leg flexed, then cross the right foot over the left knee, into four position.

Form:
Grab the right knee with the left hand and pull the knee toward the head and toward the right shoulder. Hold the stretch for 15 seconds, then repeat for the opposite side.

SACROILLIAC SQUAT STRETCH

Emphasis:
Middle gluteals and sacroilliac joint.

Position:
Stand with the feet shoulder width apart, slightly turned out, and your arms out in front.

Form:
Squat down as low as possible, rounding your back to maintain your balance at the bottom of the squat.

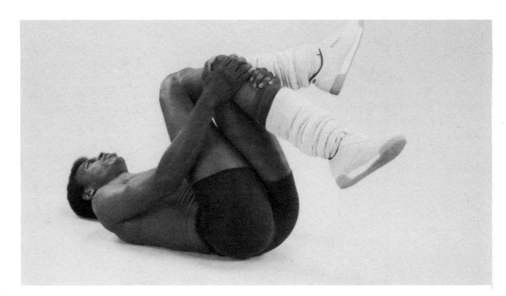

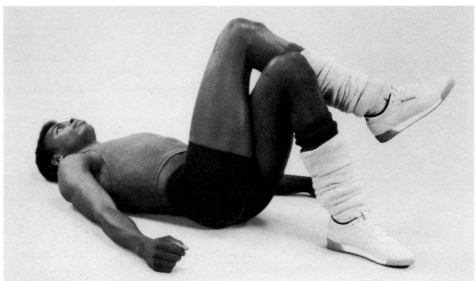

FOURTH POSITION GLUTEAL STRETCH

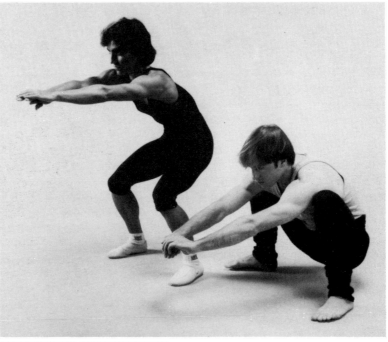

SACROILLIAC SQUAT STRETCH

PSOAS STRETCH

Emphasis:
Psoas muscle. **CAUTION!** People with lower back problems should avoid this exercise until the problem is corrected.

Position:
Start in a front position, kneeling on the left knee, with the right leg fully extended to the right side.

Form:
Slowly rotate the torso to the right, simultaneously arching the back. Hold and repeat for the opposite side.

ABDUCTOR STRETCH

Emphasis:
Abductors and obliques.

Position:
Lie on your side and place the right hand on the floor, supporting the outstretched body. Flex the left leg and cross it over the right, so that the left foot is in front of the right thigh or knee. The right arm pushes the body up straight, at about a 45-degree angle to the floor.

Form:
Press the right hip toward the floor, while arching up with the upper body. Hold the stretch and repeat for the opposite side.

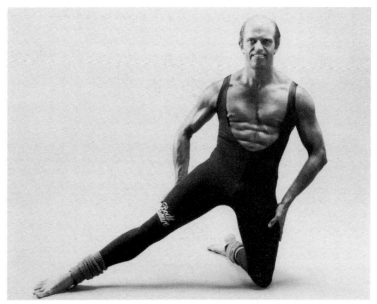

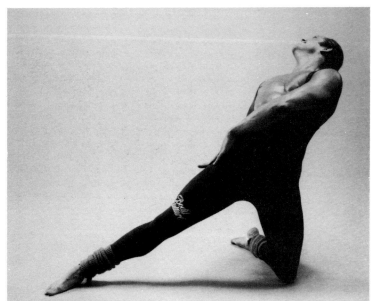

PSOAS STRETCH

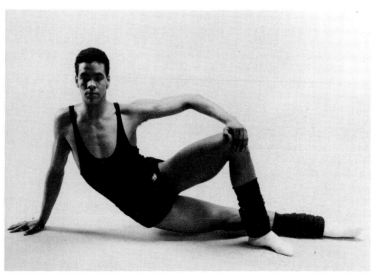

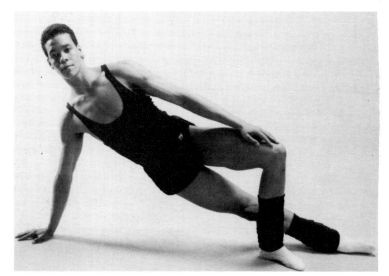

ABDUCTOR STRETCH

ABDOMINALS

ABDOMINALS

CAUTION! People with back problems must not arch too much in the abdominal stretches.

LYING SIDE POSE

Emphasis:
Abdominal muscles.

Position:
Lie on your left side, arms and legs stretched out.

Form:
Simply arch the back, reaching back with the arms and legs.

STANDING ABDOMINAL STRETCH

Emphasis:
Abdominal muscles.

Position:
Place the feet shoulder width apart. Lift the chest up and back slightly.

Form:
Pull the front pelvis down slightly and stretch the abdominals by pulling the chest higher.
NOTE: If you are feeling this stretch in the lower back, you are arching too much or pushing the hips too far forward. This stretch is accomplished by lifting the chest up.

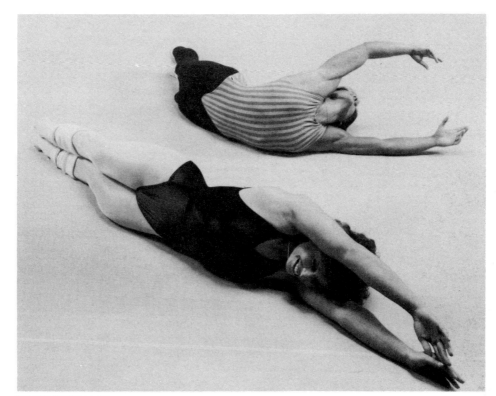

LYING SIDE POSE

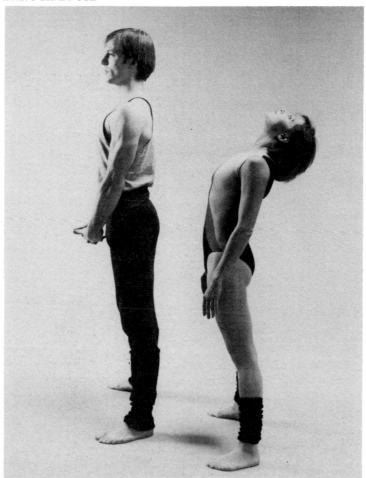

STANDING ABDOMINAL STRETCH

171

COBRA STRETCH

Emphasis:
Abdominal muscles.

Position:
Start on all fours and slowly press the hips toward the floor.

Form:
Arch the back slightly. Take a deep breath and push the stomach out. Raise the chest up. Hold for 15 seconds.

SIDES

OVERHEAD SIDE REACH

Emphasis:
Obliques and latissimus dorsi, unilaterally.

Position:
Stand with your feet a little more than shoulder width apart and your left arm over your head. Reach up, stretching that side of the ribcage.

Form:
Bend laterally to the right and reach a little more with the left arm. Repeat for the opposite side.

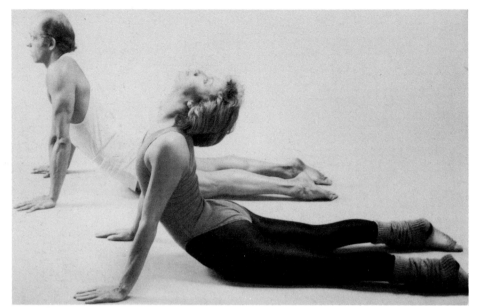

COBRA STRETCH

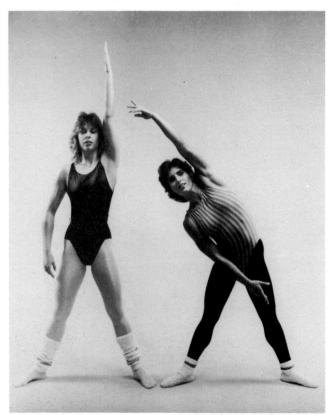

OVERHEAD SIDE REACH

172

TRIANGLE

Emphasis:
Obliques.

Position:
Stand with your feet wide apart. Bend forward and twist to the right. Grab the right foot with the left hand.

Form:
Raise the right arm straight up and pull with the left arm, keeping the head in line with the shoulders. Do not look back. Hold the stretch for 15 seconds, then repeat for the opposite side.

SPLIT SIDE STRETCH

Emphasis:
Obliques and latissimus dorsi.

Position:
Sit with the legs spread as far apart as is comfortable. Grab the right heel with the right hand, bending laterally to the side to do so.

Form:
Raise the left hand up and over, and reach out and pull with the right hand. Hold the stretch for 15 seconds, then repeat for the opposite side.

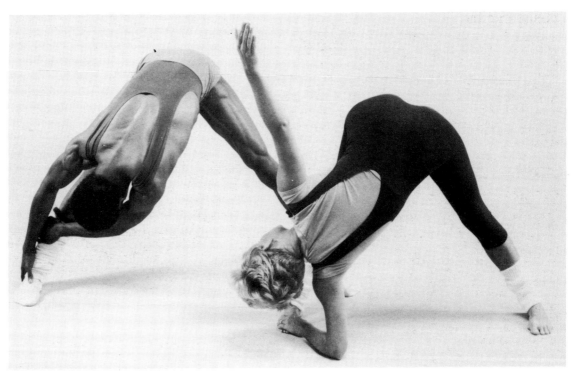

TRIANGLE

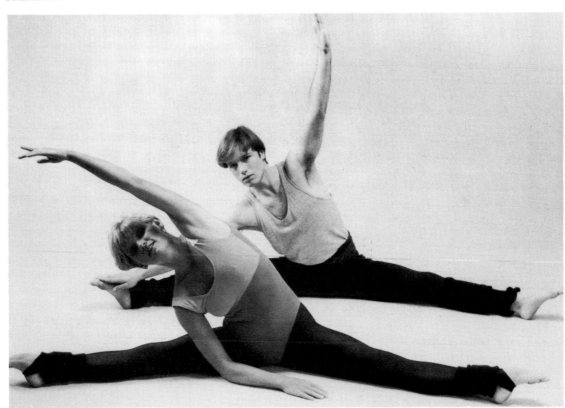

SPLIT SIDE STRETCH

GROIN

SITTING IN SECOND POSITION

Emphasis:
Adductors (groin).

Position:
Sit in second position. Bend the knees and bring the soles of the feet together in front of you. Pull the feet in with your hands, as close as possible to the body.

Form:
Hold the feet with both hands and use your elbows to press the knees toward the floor.

SIDE LUNGE

Emphasis:
Adductors.

Position:
Stand with the feet twice shoulder width apart. Bend the torso forward, parallel to the floor, and support your weight on outstretched arms. The feet are turned out.

Form:
Slowly bend the left leg and adjust the hand position to maintain the torso parallel to the floor. Keep the line of the thigh and the line of the foot in the same direction. Press the knee out and press the hip toward the floor. Hold the stretch for 15 seconds. Repeat for the opposite side.

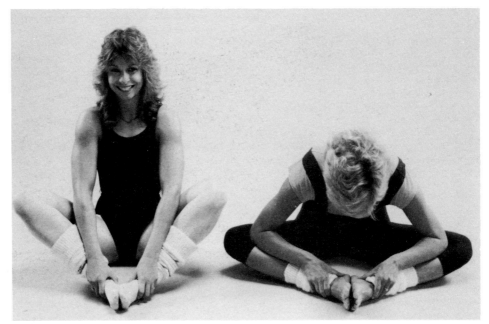

SITTING IN SECOND POSITION

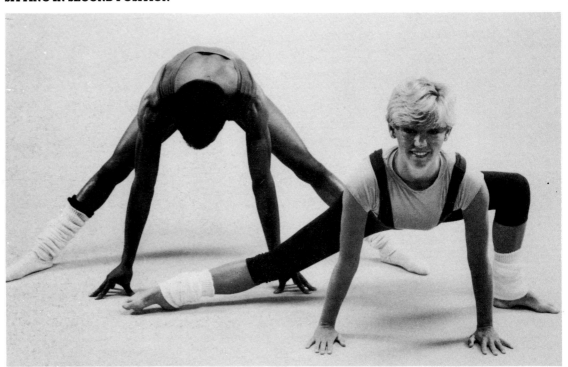

SIDE LUNGE

FRONT SPLITS

Emphasis:
Hamstring and groin.

Position:
Kneel in a hurdle position, the hands on either side for balance. Push the front heel forward.

Form:
Ease the heel forward and the groin toward the floor. Hold the stretch for 15 seconds and repeat for the opposite side. Your flexibility will determine how close you get to the ground. As a variation, you may try a straight-leg split.

SIDE SPLIT

Emphasis:
Lower adductors.

Position:
Stand with your feet twice shoulder width apart, in a natural turnout. Bend forward from the waist and support the body with outstretched arms.

Form:
Slowly inch the feet further apart, until you reach maximum stretch.

Variation:
Arch the back slightly and press the chest toward the floor. Hold the stretch for 15 seconds. Extremely flexible people will be able to put the chest on the floor with their legs fully outstretched in the split position.

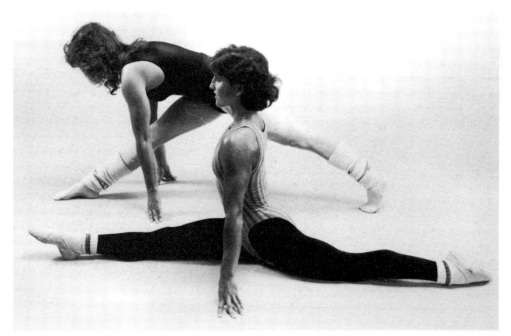

FRONT SPLITS

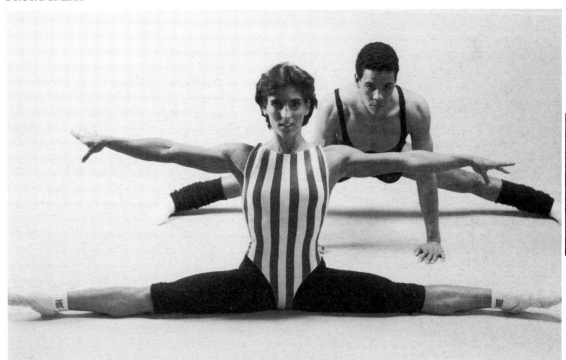

SIDE SPLIT

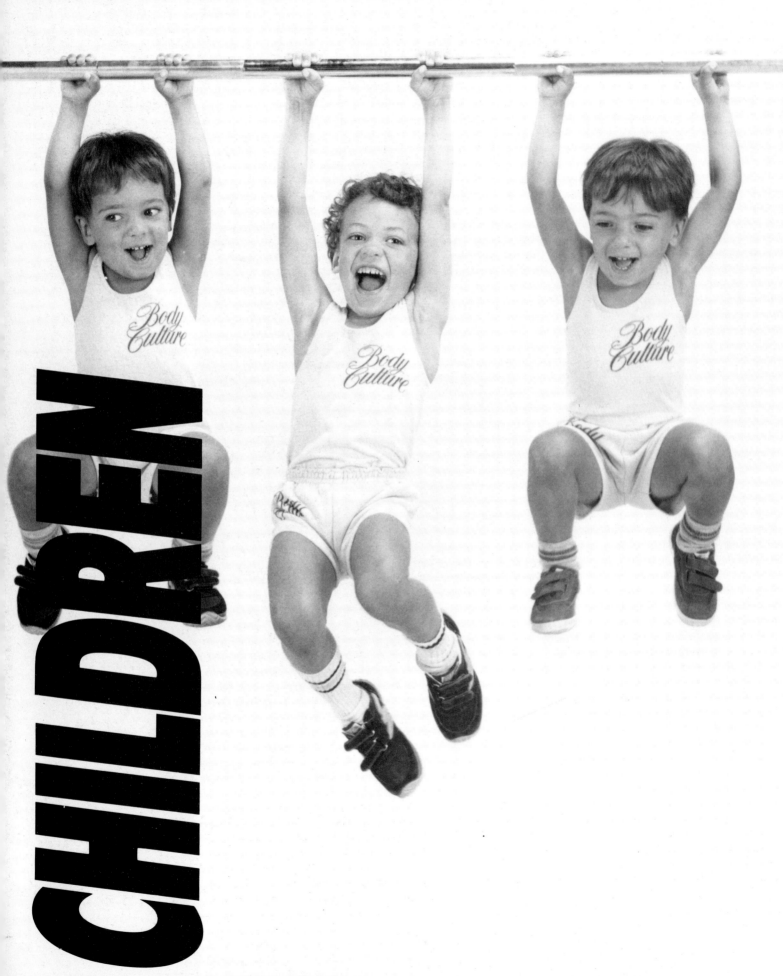

CHILDREN

Close observation of your children will reveal that both energy levels and irritability are related to diet. A high level of sugar in the diet can produce emotional and attitudinal highs and lows – the child can ride a biochemical roller coaster all day long. By introducing more complex carbohydrates into the child's diet and reducing the amount of simple sugars, a parent can give his child a more consistent and manageable energy level.

Parents must be particular about their children's food intake. I suggest some simple food rules in planning diets for growing bodies:

No refined sugar.

No white flour.

Moderate amounts of saturated (animal) fats.

Plenty of vegetables – including raw vegetables daily.

Fruit every day.

No commercial soda pop.

No candy.

Don't overcook food.

Water down sweet fruit juices.

No junk food.

Should children be encouraged to exercise at an early age?

Many parents and patients express concern about when their children should begin physical training. In answering such questions, I always give the example of my sons, who are typical, young, healthy and active boys.

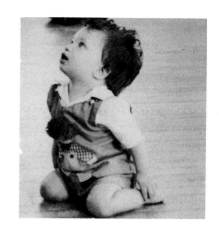

I certainly don't need to encourage them to exercise. In fact, the only problem my wife and I experience is in getting them to slow down long enough to eat or to sleep. The amount of activity they get through play – and which is similar for most of the children on our street – is sufficient for their early development.

An important aspect of play for a child's future development is his freedom to experiment with growing physical abilities in a safe environment. It is important to reach for one's potential at every age. I never refuse to let my boys try something new, unless I consider it dangerous. My definition of "safe" activities may be broader than that of other parents, but this is because I have carefully watched the growth of motor skills in my sons and know what they can handle.

All my sons began swimming lessons when they were only six months old and they are all comfortable and confident in the water. They learn motor skills plus organization through team play in soccer, hockey and T-ball. My 4-year-old races bicycle moto-cross in the age 7-and-under class and handles himself very well. My advice is to make it safe, and let them reach and develop.

As for specific muscle development, my boys like to be with me when I am working around the house or exercising in my gym on the third floor. I purchased a set of light weights – 2.5, 5 and 7 pounds – with which they can imitate the various exercises I am performing. This is voluntary.

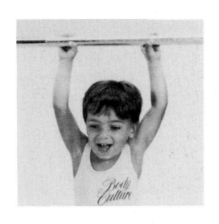

*T*he kids may pick up a weight and try to copy my form, but if it is too difficult or too heavy, they are free to go off running or cycling. If they want to exercise, I help them and make it safe for them. However, I don't force them into training if they are not interested, because this could have a discouraging effect in later years. If exercise isn't fun for children when they are young, they will later display a subconscious aversion to it. The emphasis must be on fun.

*C*hildren shouldn't be pushed into weight training at too young an age because the growth plates on their bones have not yet fused. Boys usually don't finish this process years until ages 16 to 18. Girls mature physically one or two years earlier than boys.

*I*f children are required to use maximum effort to lift heavy weights before the growth plates have fused, the plates may be forced out of place by the excessive stress, stunting the growth or causing uneven growth.

*I*f children do show an early interest in weight training, make certain that they use only very light weights and spend most of their time concentrating on form.

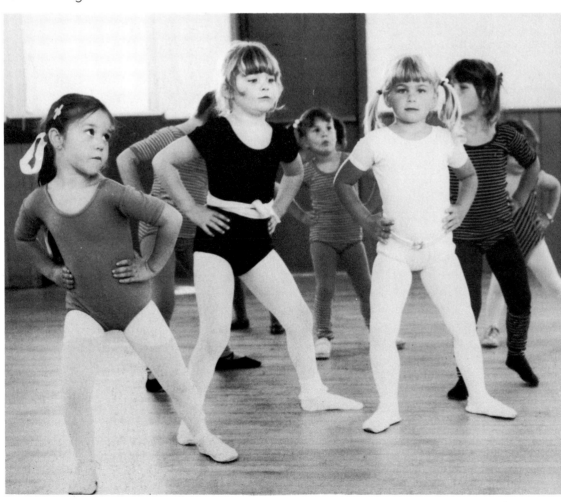

Structured exercise classes and organized gym programs are a valuable tool for children in learning to control and direct their energies. My sister teaches aerobics for children from ages 4 to 7. It takes a few classes to get the children to join in, then a few more to perform the exercises properly, until it becomes a fun event. Again, the classes incorporate basic elements of play – jogging and jumping, rolling and twisting, stretching and curling up, clapping and waving their arms about – to stimulate the use of all different muscle groups.

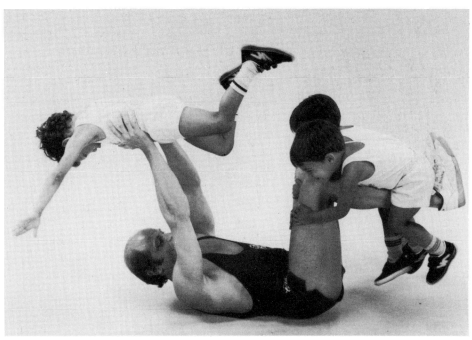

One thing parents should monitor closely in their children is body fat. In Victorian days, a chubby infant was considered a healthy infant, the embodiment of a family's prosperity. We know now that this is actually an unhealthy state, taxing the young heart and clogging up the child's arteries.

The number of fat cells a person will have in life is determined by the age of three. If a child is obese before that time, that child will have a large number of fat cells for his entire life and will find it more difficult to lose weight when he gets older.

The way to control a youngster's weight gain is, of course, through diet. Kids would eat ice cream and junk food all day long if parents permitted it. It is up to parents to provide the proper foods for their children.

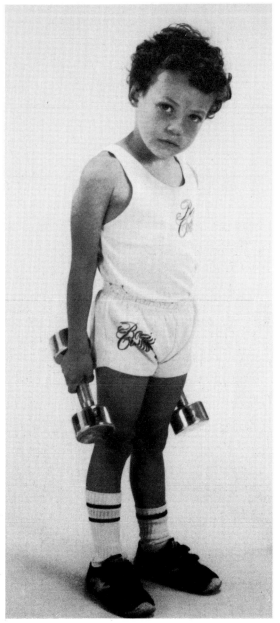

BACK CARE

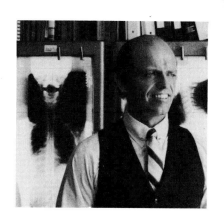

It may sound unbelievable, but some 80 per cent of the population has back problems. Almost no one goes through life without suffering back pain at some time. Therefore, it is necessary to include a section in this exercise book on cautions, precautions and care for a very common problem.

Years ago, it was thought that lifting caused most back problems and that running, exercise and weightlifting were almost certain to give you lingering pain. We know now that these activities can be done safely. It is when they are incorrectly performed that they exaggerate or exacerbate an existing back problem or exploit some latent mechanical or structural weakness in the back.

The predisposing factor present in most people, that makes them susceptible to back problems from exercise, is what chiropractors have identified for years as subluxations. A subluxation in the spine is a misalignment or disrelationship of adjacent vertebrae. This can produce pressure on the nerves coming through openings between the vertebrae or interfere with mobility of the spine.

A subluxation can exist in a subclinical state, meaning that no noticeable symptoms are evident. Then, a sudden movement, an incorrectly performed exercise, a heavy load lifted improperly – even a violent sneeze – can aggravate the subluxation. It produces pain; sometimes functional symptoms develop.

Understand that exercises performed correctly don't cause these problems in a properly aligned spine, but can be a catalyst to the symptoms when there is an existing predisposition (subluxation).

PREVENTION

The key to avoiding back pain, as in other areas of health, lies in prevention. Have a chiropractor examine your spine for any indications of subluxations which could make you vulnerable to future injury. If any are detected, take the time to get them corrected before they give you problems.

The best method for avoiding injury during exercise is to use proper form always. The sections of this book on weight training, aerobics and stretching all include detailed explanations of the proper form for executing each exercise. Follow the explanations on form fully, paying attention to every detail – including the caution advisories. They are

here to help you achieve maximum results, while preventing back injuries.

WHAT TO DO WHEN IT HURTS

If a back injury occurs during your exercise program, what should you do?

1. Keep warm. If the clothes you are wearing are sweaty, change them and bundle up.

2. Go straight to a back-care specialist. The sooner you get professional chiropractic help, the faster your recovery will be.

3. Understand what happened, how to get it corrected, and – most important – how to avoid the recurrence of the same injury. Don't rush back into the same exercises without checking form and don't resume training at the same level. Work your way back gradually.

Once professional treatment has begun and you are pain-free enough to start exercising, consult the following list of exercises and stretches to speed up rehabilitation and to ensure your ability to maintain the spinal adjustments you have received. The exercises are arranged in the order most people can perform them as they recover from back injury.

BACK REHABILITATION

Rehabilitation of a back injury requires not only the correction of a subluxation, but the strengthening of supporting muscles. Only after this has been accomplished should you consider resuming your previous exercise program. Resume the exercises slowly – at a lower gradient level than before, with less weight and fewer repetitions than you were performing at the time of injury. In aerobic activities, drop back one level.

Be meticulous about form.

Heed your professional's advice when he cautions you about particular activities. A back injury has a certain similarity to a sprained ankle: once severely injured, it can tend to recur and become your "Achilles heel" in physical activity.

Therefore, it is necessary to maintain the integrity of the spine after it has been corrected. Regular checkups, along with a form-conscious exercise program for abdominal and back muscles will help prevent recurrences.

BACK EXERCISES

EGG ROLL

Emphasis:
To massage the back.

Position:
Lie on your back and bring both knees up toward the chest. Clasp you hands just below the knees and flex the neck and head toward the chest.

Form:
Roll back and forth on your back. This exercise loosens tight muscles and limbers the back when people are unable to do much more. This should not be painful. If it is, you are not ready to start any exercise.

CAT STRETCH

Emphasis:
Stretches and strengthens the abdominal and erector spinae muscles.

Position:
Kneel on all fours, hands palms down, just a little wider than shoulder width apart, and knees shoulder width apart.

Form:
Lower the abdomen and chest toward the floor and raise the buttocks toward the ceiling, contracting the lower back muscles and stretching the abdominal muscles. Next, lower the buttocks and head while raising the back into an arch, stretching the back and contracting the abdominals.

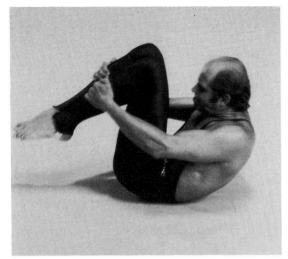
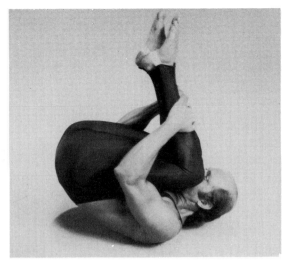

EGG ROLL

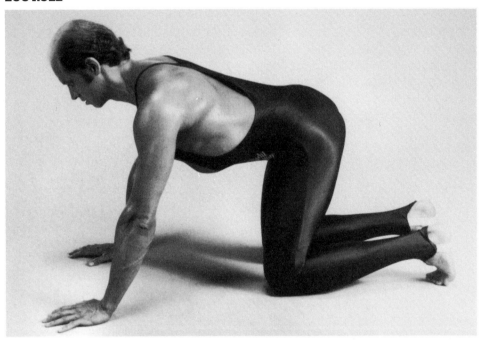

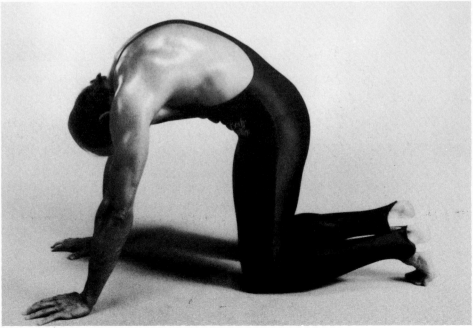

CAT STRETCH

182

PELVIC TILT

Emphasis:
Abdominals, buttocks and erector spinae.

Position:
Lie supine on the floor with legs bent and feet flat. This will flatten the lower back.

Form:
Tilt the pelvis forward (toward the ceiling) by contracting the abdominals and buttocks. This will lift the lower buttocks off the floor slightly. Then, relax the abdominals and buttocks and contract the erector spinae muscles to rock the pelvis backwards (toward the floor). This exercise may also be done standing, with the back against the wall and the knees slightly bent.

KNEES TO CHEST

Emphasis:
Strengthens quadriceps, abdominals and iliopsoas and stretches the hamstrings.

Position:
Lie supine on the floor, legs flat.

Form:
Bring one knee up toward the chest and return it to the floor. Alternate legs. Stretch as shown and described in knees-to-chest exercise in the stretch section of the text.

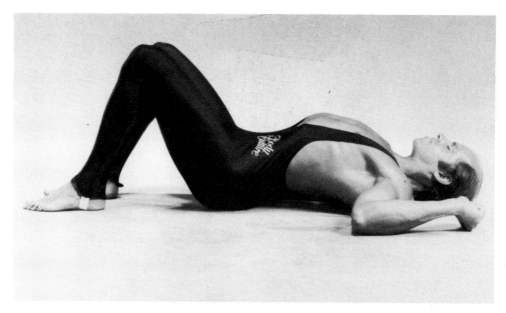

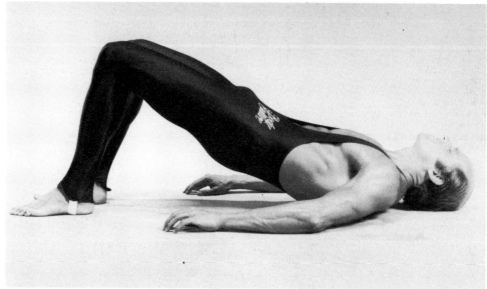

PELVIC TILT

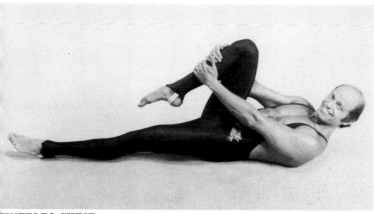

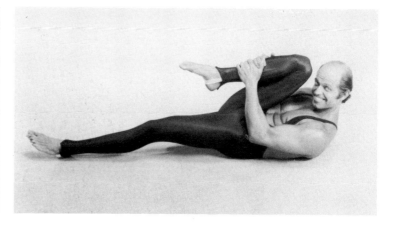

KNEES TO CHEST

183

SIDE-TO-SIDE KNEE PULL

Emphasis:
Erector spinae, obliques, buttocks and abductors.

Position:
Lie supine and bend the knees up toward the chest until the thighs are a little past vertical. The arms are outstretched for balance. Keep the knees together.

Form:
Slowly lower the knees to one side, maintaining balance (shoulders square to floor). Lift and repeat, lowering to opposite side.

TWISTS

Emphasis:
Erector spinae, obliques and abdominals.

Position:
Stand erect, with the feet 24 to 26 inches apart. Bend the knees slightly, with the arms extended horizontally.

Form:
Slowly twist to one side, keeping the head, shoulders and arms square. Go as far as you can, comfortably. Slowly return to starting position and repeat to the other side. You may also perform the exercise with the legs straight, allowing a further rotation by permitting more pelvic movement (as shown).

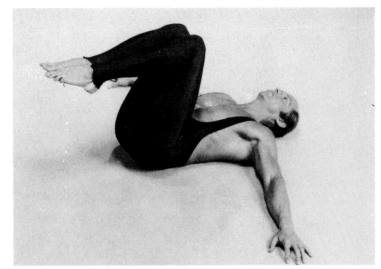

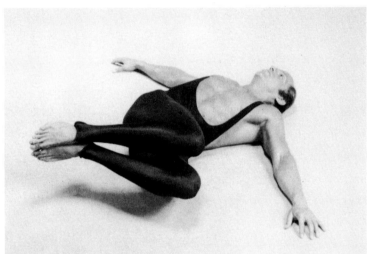

SIDE-TO-SIDE KNEE PULL

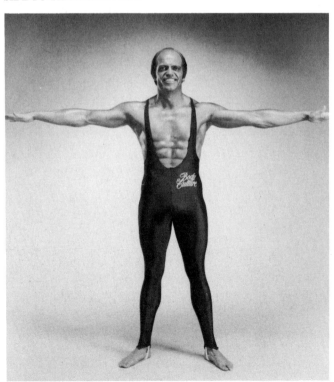

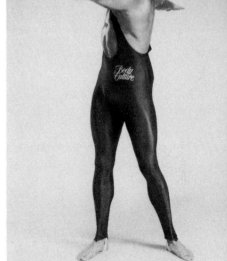

TWISTS

184

SIDE BENDS

Emphasis:
Obliques, latissimus dorsi and erector spinae.

Position:
Stand with feet shoulder width apart, hands at the sides.

Form:
Lean laterally to the right side, sliding the right hand down the side of the leg. Contract the oblique muscle on the right side and stretch the oblique muscle on the left side. Slowly return to starting position and repeat for the opposite side.

LEG EXTENSIONS

Emphasis:
Erector spinae, buttocks, hamstrings.

Position:
Lie face down on the floor, arms up and to the side for balance.

Form:
Raise the right leg up, keeping it straight. Use the erector spinae and gluteal muscles to raise the leg as high as possible. Keeping the pelvis flat on the floor, contract the erector spinae muscles and hold for a slow count of three. Return the leg almost to the floor, then raise it again, slowly. Repeat 10 times for each side. This exercise also may be done raising both legs at the same time, or may be done in a kneeling position, with the upper body supported over the side of a bed or box.

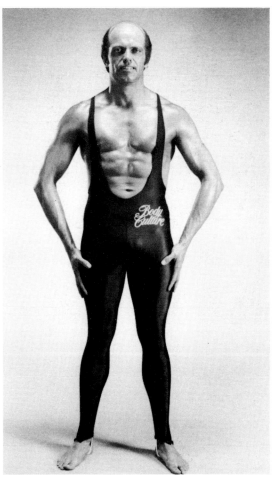 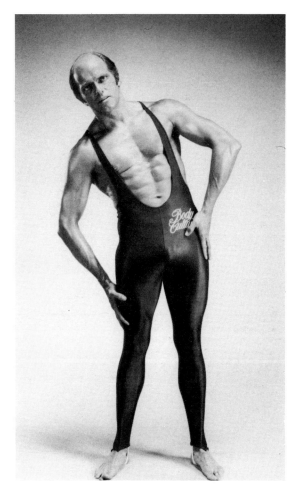

SIDE BENDS

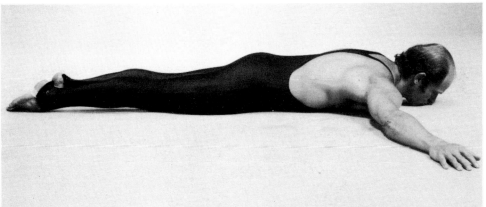

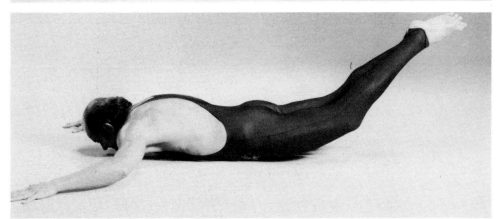

LEG EXTENSIONS

185

EXTENSIONS

Emphasis:
Erector spinae (lower back) and cervical extensors (back of the neck).

Position:
Lie face down on the floor, arms at your sides, legs out straight.

Form:
Slowly contract the erector spinae muscles to raise the upper body off the floor. The neck and head are extended as well. Raise as high as you can, comfortably, and hold for a slow count of three before lowering. The exercise may also be done with the upper body hanging over the edge of a bed or bench, while a partner holds your heels (see weight training section). The arm position may also be varied for added resistance.

DEEP SQUAT

Emphasis:
Middle gluteals and sacroilliac joint.

Position:
Stand with the feet shoulder width apart, slightly turned out, and your arms out in front.

Form:
Squat down as low as possible, rounding your back to maintain your balance at the bottom of the squat.

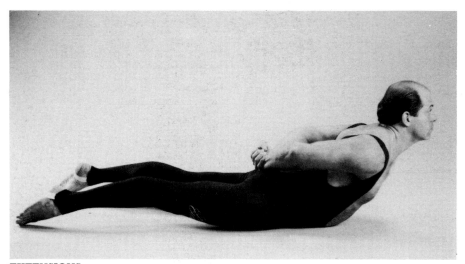

EXTENSIONS

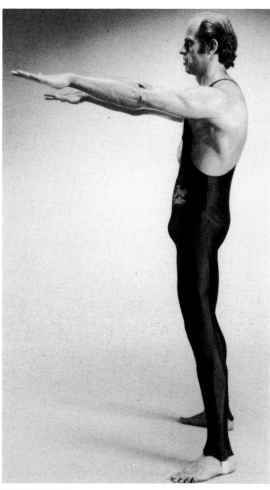
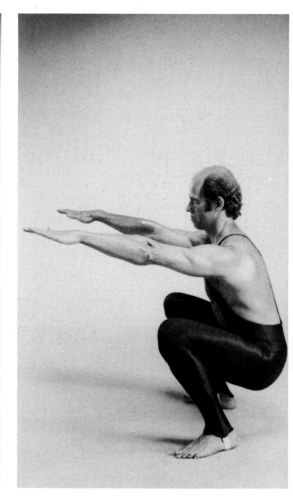

DEEP SQUAT

TOE TOUCHES

Emphasis:
Hamstrings, buttocks, erector spinae (lower back).

Position:
Stand erect, with the arms hanging down, the feet slightly apart for balance.

Form:
Bend forward, slowly sliding the hands down the front of the legs. Go down as far as comfortable and hold, then slowly raise the body back to the upright position. This exercise may also be done from a sitting position.

CAUTION! This is the last exercise in this series and should only be done once free of pain. Even then, execute it slowly and do not bounce the stretch.
The next step in a rehabilitation program is to strengthen the abdominal muscles, since these provide musch support for the back.

ABDOMINAL CRUNCHES

Emphasis:
Abdominal muscles and front neck muscles.

Position:
Lie supine, with the legs bent and the arms folded over the chest. If you are more advanced, the hand position is beside the hips.

Form:
Slowly contract the abdominal muscles to raise the head and shoulders and upper back off the floor. Hold for a count of three and squeeze the abdominals, then release and lower – but do not let the head touch the floor. Repeat.
See the weight training and aerobic sections for more varieties of abdominal exercises.

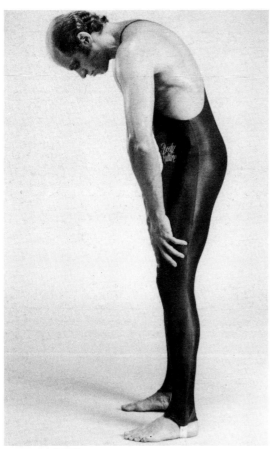
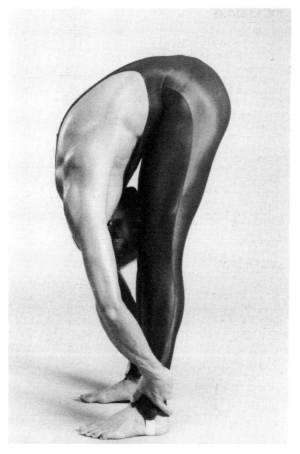

TOE TOUCHES

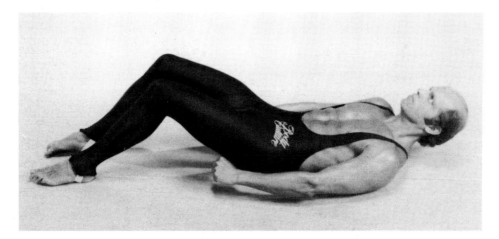

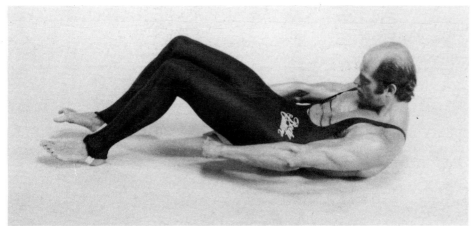

ABDOMINAL CRUNCHES

187

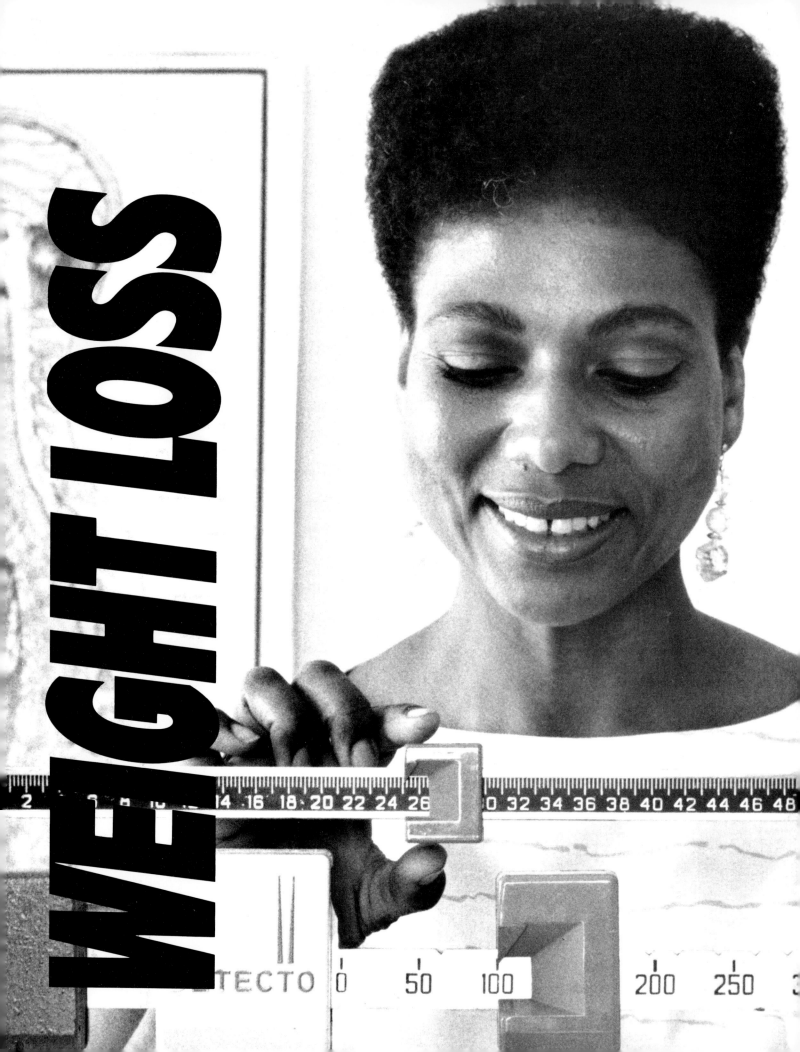

WEIGHT LOSS

TECTO   0   50   100   200   250

WEIGHT LOSS

*T*he loss of weight through the loss of body fat should be simple mathematics: decrease the amount of food going into the body (diet) and increase the amount of energy expended (exercise). But for most people, it is not quite so easy.

*T*he knowledge that an excess accumulation of 3,500 calories (that is, 3,500 calories more than you burn up) is equal to a pound of accumulated body fat does not tell you how to get the weight off and keep it off.

*T*he diet, lifestyle changes and exercise programs used in the Body Culture diet are designed to address the plateaus and stumbling blocks often encountered when a person tries to lose weight.

*T*his very chapter is the result of requests by my wife and five other new mothers who were all having difficulty losing weight accumulated during pregnancy and breast feeding. The following program incorporates exercises from the book the diets used in our clinic.

DIET

*T*he objective of our program is to teach a new lifestyle of proper nutritional habits and regular exercise to enable the participants to lose weight, then maintain the loss. We have found that a number of people who lose weight on any number of special diets have a tendency to put the weight right back on, as soon as the dieting period is finished. We call this the yo-yo effect.

*T*his occurs because, although there has temporarily been a substantial reduction of calorie intake, there has been no effort made to alter the lifestyle. These people haven't been taught how to design their own dietary and exercise programs. They revert to old habits and gain the weight back again. The goal of the Body Culture diet is more than just a number on a scale. Our end product is meant to be a new person who has achieved their desired weight and fitness levels, and who has gained the knowledge and ability to regulate themselves thereafter.

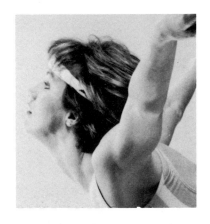

*S*pace limitations do not permit the inclusion of the entire Body Culture diet program, but we present this condensed version in step-by-step form.

1. The participants were weighed and measured, with both a tape measure and a set of fat calipers. The calipers give measurement of fat calibrated pinch-test. The participants also agreed to have pictures taken for before-and-after comparisons, a courageous step for people who are overweight.

2. A complete health history was taken and a dietary questionnaire was filled out. Any health problems were noted and attended to. It is very difficult to concentrate on diet and exercise if you are unhealthy. Detrimental habits – such as smoking – were also addressed.

3. The participants made a six-month committment to their diets and exercise programs and agreed to follow our recommendations.

4. An instructional package was issued with the general rules and explanations of the program.

5. The first diet was a seven-day cleansing diet, designed to clean out the bulk accumulated in the intestines. A sluggish digestive system tends to inhibit the effect and diminish the results obtained from a weight loss diet.
Participants lost between four and seven pounds on this seven-day elimination plan.

6. The participants signed up for aerobics and stretch classes, under the direction of Al Greene at Body Alive. The minimum requirement was three classes per week. They began with technique classes, then progressed to stretch classes to prepare their bodies for real work. They then moved from beginners' classes to the intermediate level after one or two months.

7. The second diet recommended to them was a planned one-week diet which allowed 1,000 calories per day. This was repeated weekly for one month.

8. Weekly meetings were arranged to distribute new materials, answer questions and handle any problems encountered. It might also be noted that these meetings of the participants also brought them together as a peer group. They could offer support and encouragement to one another, as well as provide pressure to stick to what the group was doing – keep up one's end, so to speak.

9. The first step in the lifestyle change involved having the participants research the calories, fat, protein, sugar, carbohydrate and sodium content of all the foods on the 1,000-calorie diet.

10. At the end of the first month, weight and measurements were reevaluated for comparison.

11. Each person was given some special vitamins and minerals to help facilitate the burning of fat and to help eliminate excess water.

12. For homework, each of the participants was required to design a full day's meals (totalling 1,000 calories), using the principles of the Body Culture diet.

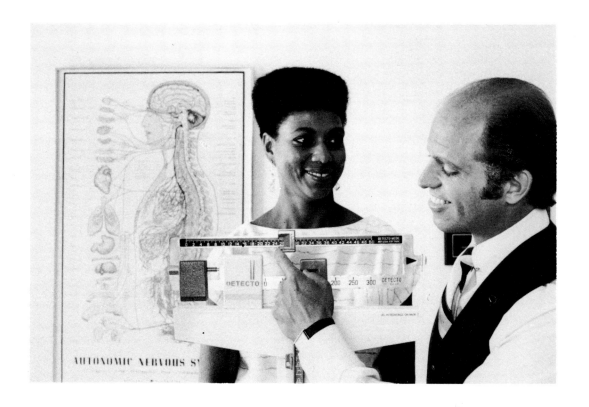

13. Over the next month the participants helped design more than 30 different recipes for a greater variety of meal selection.

14. Some of the subjects increased the intensity of their workouts and advanced to the intermediate level of aerobics. A few increased frequency of workouts to four and five times per week. This increased activity boosted the effectiveness of the program.

15. A third set of measurements was taken. This was an important step, because a few participants were feeling disappointed when their weight seemed to level off (a sticking point). Both the tape measure and the caliper skinfold measurements confirmed that they were, indeed, losing fat. The reason weight loss appeared to stop was that they were working hard enough to be putting on muscle while burning off fat.

16. A herbal combination was introduced to further cleanse the bowels.

17. Some individual changes were implemented at this point, to deal with particular problem areas.

18. When most of the participants reached their weight goals, we introduced a weight-training program which could be followed at home.

19. By this time, all participants were able to design their own diets, based on Body Culture principles and on their own specific requirements.

*T*he results of the first three months of the program are documented here for you with the before-and-after pictures. The key to the Body Culture diet's success is that it is combined with the exercises described in this book.

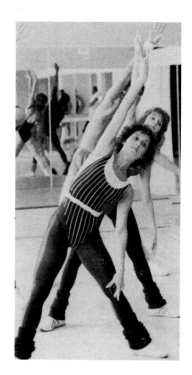

Joni Turner, 37.

Mother of four children, ages 4, 2 1/2 (twins) and 14 months. Reason for being overweight – pregnancies. Started Body Culture program at 145 pounds in April and reduced to 128 by July, trimming waist measurement by more than three inches and hips by more than five inches.

"The best diet I have ever been on. I did not have to starve to lose weight. Doing the aerobics gave me more energy and exercising also made me more patient with my children. I feel good and my husband finds me more attractive."

Weight Loss Program

	Before	After
Weight	145	128
Waist	30½″	27″
Hips	42″	36½″
Thighs	24½″	22″
Chest	36″	34½″

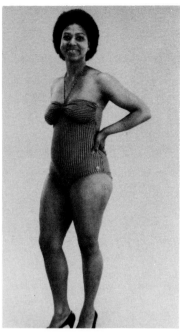
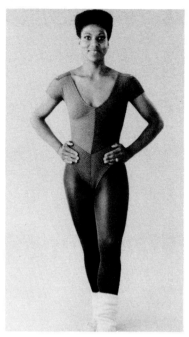

Mairead Rooney, 28.

Mother of children aged 2 1/2 years and 7 months. Reason for being overweight – pregnancy and lack of disciplined eating habits. Weight dropped from 135 1/2 pounds to 123 3/4 pounds, losing two inches off the waist.

"The program was a lot of hard work. I still have to firm up and lose four more pounds, but it got easier as time went on and the achievements gave me incentive to continue."

Weight Loss Program

	Before	After
Weight	135	123
Waist	31″	29″
Hips	38″	36″
Thighs	36″	33½″
Chest	36″	35″

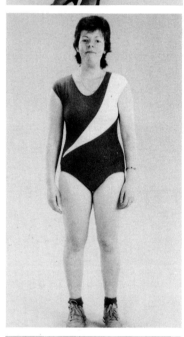
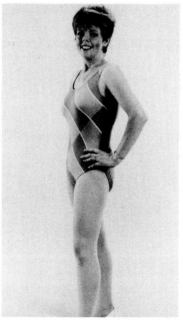

Maureen Fitzgerald, 34.

Mother of children aged 3 1/2 years and 21 months. Reason for being overweight – childbearing, lack of exercise and over-eating to compensate for fatigue.

"The diet has changed my approach to food so that now I feel confident I can keep my weight under control. My original goal was 130 pounds but I achieved 124! I look forward to exercise for the first time in years. An added bonus is that I have no more lower back pain."

Weight Loss Program

	Before	After
Weight	158	124
Waist	35″	28″
Hips	43″	36½″
Thighs	25″	21″
Chest	42½″	35″
Arms	11½″	10½″

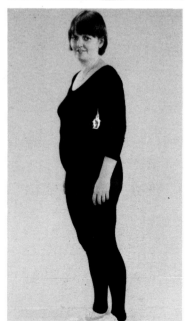
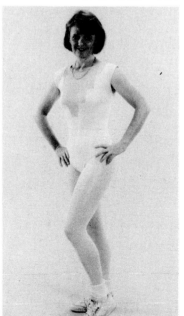

Gail Simpson, 28.

Cashier and mother of children aged 4 1/2 years and nine months. Reasons for overweight – overeating, especially when feeling tense or hyper. Program included four aerobics and four stretch classes per week, as well as running.

"Diet and exercise firmed me up and brought my weight back to 110 pounds. It was tough but worth it. I feel good and hope to continue."

Weight Loss Program

	Before	After
Weight	120	113
Waist	27½"	25½"
Hips	36"	35"
Thighs	22"	20¼"
Chest	33"	32¼"
Arms	10½"	10½"

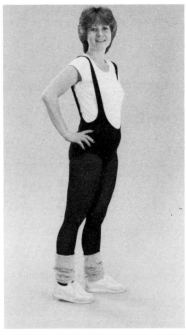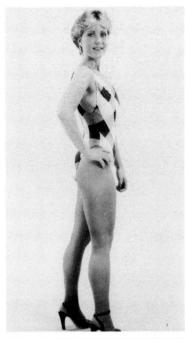

Francis Kupka, 37

Tapestry weaver and medical illustrator. She became overweight initially because of pregnancy, and then began to overeat compulsively because of the stresses of having both a career and family.

"Losing weight is definitely easier when exercise is included. Exercise increased my self esteem and energy level. Another essential part of the program was the supervision Dr. Turner gave me concerning diet and nutrition. It helped me stick to the program."

Weight Loss Program

	Before	After
Weight	155	139
Waist	33½"	29½"
Hips	44½"	37"
Thighs	26"	23"
Chest	36½"	37"
Arms	12"	11"

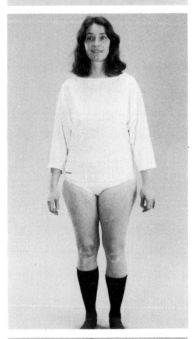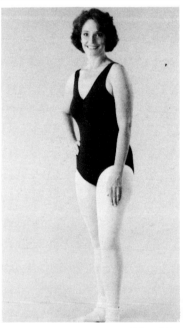

Barb O'Bieirne, 31

Graphic artist and mother, I became overweight by just falling into the bad habit of overeating and not being active enough.

"The body culture program is one that I can live with. Exercise has now become a permanent part of my family's life. In any weight loss program, exercise is essential. Psychologically, as well as physically, it makes the diet easier to follow."

Weight Loss Program

	Before	After
Weight	175	150
Waist	37"	29"
Hips	44"	40"
Thighs	25"	22"
Chest	40½"	38"
Arms	12"	10½"

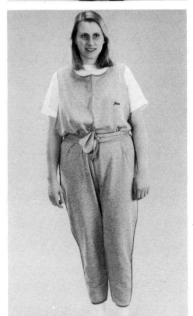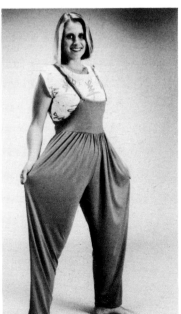

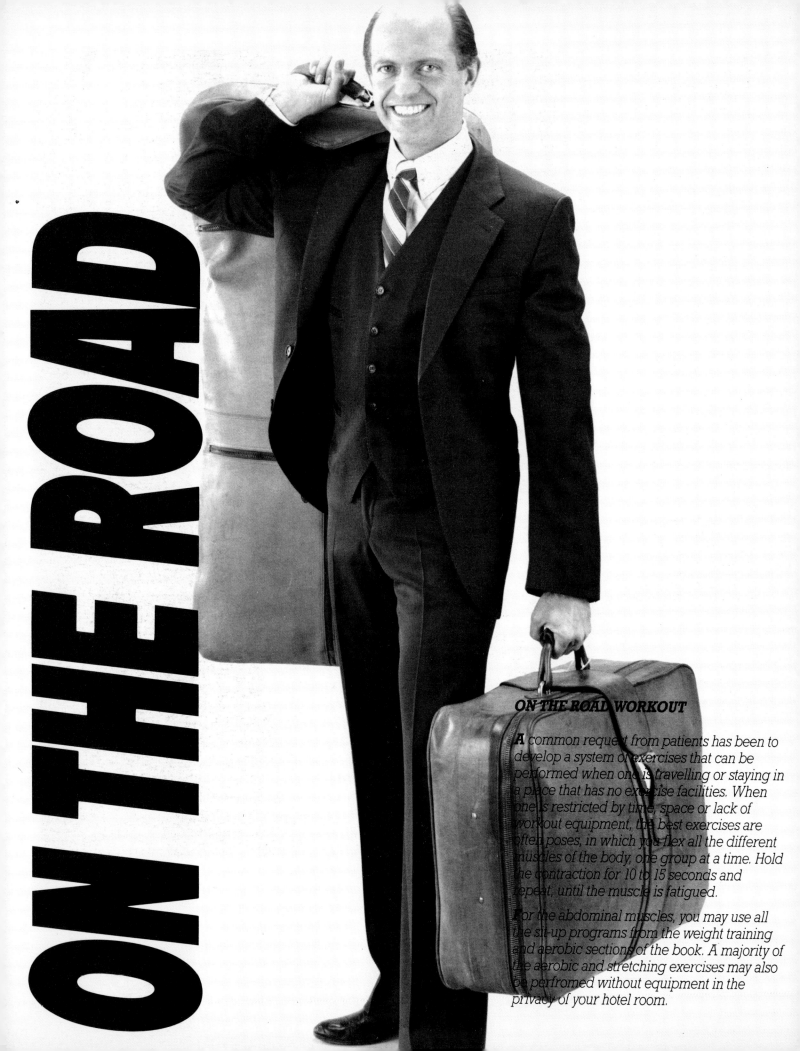

ON THE ROAD

ON THE ROAD WORKOUT

A common request from patients has been to develop a system of exercises that can be performed when one is travelling or staying in a place that has no exercise facilities. When one is restricted by time, space or lack of workout equipment, the best exercises are often poses, in which you flex all the different muscles of the body, one group at a time. Hold the contraction for 10 to 15 seconds and repeat, until the muscle is fatigued.

For the abdominal muscles, you may use all the sit-up programs from the weight training and aerobic sections of the book. A majority of the aerobic and stretching exercises may also be perfromed without equipment in the privacy of your hotel room.

WARM-UP

Flex each muscle for two seconds and relax. Repeat this three times, starting with the upper leg, through to the calf. It is best to face a mirror to observe the contracting muscles.

LEGS

Emphasis:
Quadriceps, hamstrings, calves.

Form (1):
For the front pose, stand with your feet six to 12 inches apart and bend them slightly. Tighten the quadriceps (front thighs), hamstrings (back of the upper leg) and calves, all at the same time. To flex, force the upper legs forward and out, but do not move them. Hold for 10 seconds and repeat.

Form (2):
Place one leg slightly in front of the other and extend it fully. Now, flex the quadriceps hard and hold for 10 seconds. Repeat this several times. Switch for the other leg.

Form (3):
The calf pose is performed by standing with your right leg 12 to 18 inches behind the left. Point your right foot and rest it on the floor with only the toes touching the surface. Push up from the toes to a full contraction of the calf muscle. Hold for 10 seconds, repeat and switch for the opposite side.

SHOULDERS

Emphasis:
Rear and middle deltoids.

Form: (1)
Place your hands in front of you. Grab your left wrist with your right hand and pull it over in line with the right side of the body, elbows bent at 90 degrees. Hold the hands in this position, with the right hand, while pulling your left shoulder to the left. Hold the pose for 10 seconds and repeat. Switch hands for opposite shoulder.

Emphasis:
Front deltoids.

Form: (2)
Place your hands behind your back and take the same position. The left arm will be slightly bent. Hold the left hand steady with the right, and flex the shoulder and tricep, while pulling away from the right hand. Hold for 10 seconds, repeat and switch for opposite side.

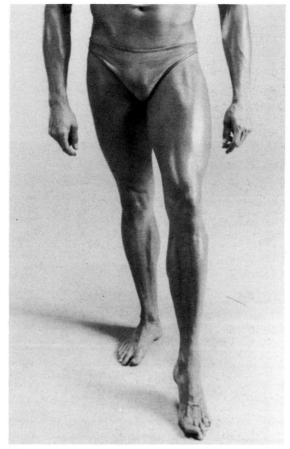
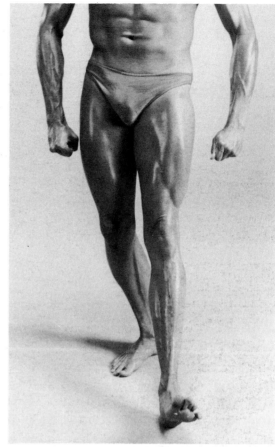

LEGS

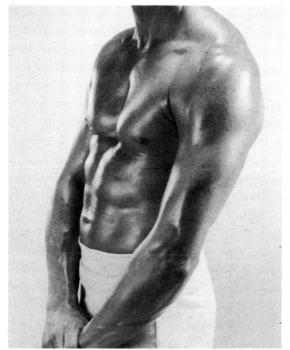
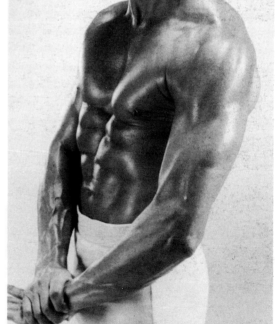

SHOULDERS

CHEST

Emphasis:
Pectorals.

Form (1):
For the hand-assisted pose, place your right hand on the left side of your chest, with the heel of the thumb against the mid-line of the pectoral muscle. Contract the left pectoral toward the center (sternum) and push gently with the right hand against the flexed pectoral. Hold for 10 seconds, repeat and switch for the opposite side. This emphasizes the midline of the pectorals.

Form (2):
Bend over slightly in the cable pull position, with the arms down and the head up. Raise the elbows up to 45 degrees and pull the arms together by flexing the pectorals (starting at the bottom of the pectorals and finishing at the top). The flex is like a wave passing through the muscle. You finish with the wrists crossed in front of you and the muscle fully flexed.

BACK

Emphasis:
Upper and lower back and latissimus dorsi.

Form (1):
The rear bicep pose stresses the upper back and latissimus. Stand with your arms up in the bicep position. Flex the muscles of the upper back by slightly pulling the shoulder blades together, but keeping the arms up and flexed as well. Also try to flare out the latissimus in this pose. It will take practice to master this one.

Form (2):
The rear pull down will work the latissimus and the middle back. Stand with your arms slightly bent over your head. Flex the latissimus and middle back and pull the arms down slowly, concentrating on flexion below the shoulder blades. Pull down until the upper arm is parallel to the floor.

ABDOMEN

Front:
Stand with one foot slightly in front of the other. Place your hand behind your head.
Contract the abdominals by sucking in the stomach slightly while contracting the rectus and obliques as well.
Once you have mastered this you can flex the quads of the leg in front.

Note:
Do not pull very hard on the back of the neck. This is for stability only.
Oblique and Serratus: Stand sideways to the mirror with one hand behind your head (Hand closest to the mirror).
Contract the serratus and obliques by bending slightly toward the mirror and pulling down and in with the above muscles.
Keep the stomach flat. Hold the flex for 10 seconds and repeat several times, then switch to the other side.

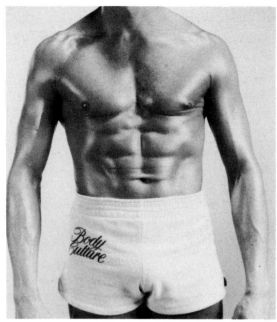 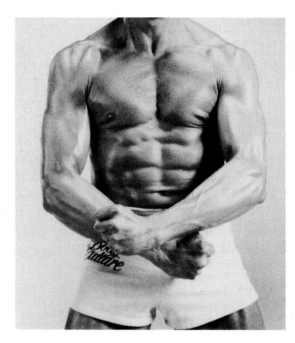

CHEST

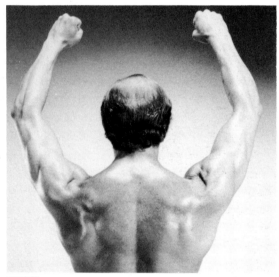 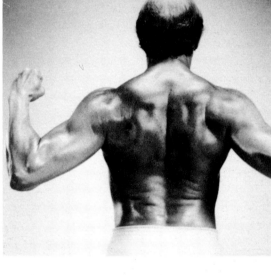

BACK

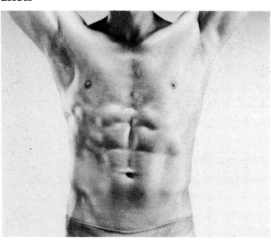 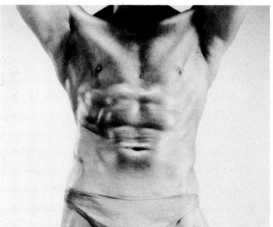

ABDOMEN

BICEPS

Emphasis:
Biceps.

Form (1):
For the double front bicep, stand with your arms up in the bicep (muscleman) pose, the upper arm parallel to the floor and elbows flexed a little more than 90 degrees. Flex as hard as you can and hold for 10 seconds. Repeat.

Form (2):
In the bicep curl, grasp your left wrist with your right hand, in front of the body. Straighten the arms. Flex the left arm while resisting with the right hand, permitting only minimal movement while exerting a maximal contraction of the bicep. Flex the arm all the way up to full contraction of the bicep. Hold for three seconds and slowly, against strong resistance from the right hand, lower it again through the negative phase. Repeat several times and switch for the opposite arm.

TRICEPS

Emphasis:
Triceps.

Form (1):
For the full extension, hang the arms down and fully extend both of them. It may help to supinate the hand, outward. Squeeze the tricep as hard as you can and hold for 10 seconds. Repeat.

Form (2):
Grasp your right wrist with your left hand, behind the back. Extend the right arm against pressure from the left hand and squeeze the tricep hard. Hold for 10 seconds, repeat and switch for the opposite side.

FOREARMS

Emphasis:
Flexors and extensors.

Form (1):
To work the flexors, begin with the right wrist cocked back or supinated and place the left palm on the right. Resisting with the left hand, flex the right wrist slowly, until it is completely flexed. Hold for three seconds and resist as you slowly extend it. Repeat and switch for the opposite wrist.

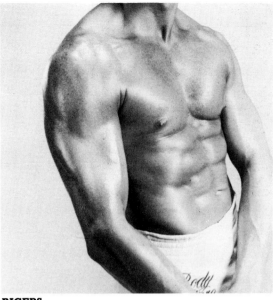
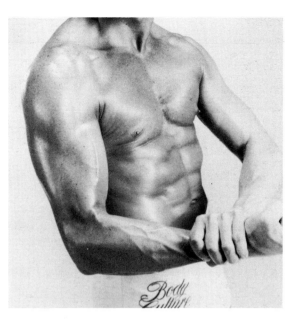

BICEPS

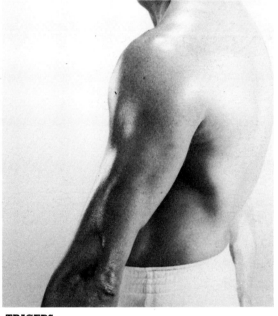
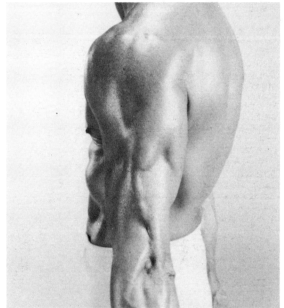

TRICEPS

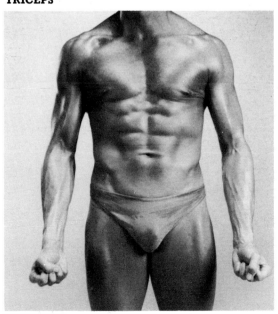
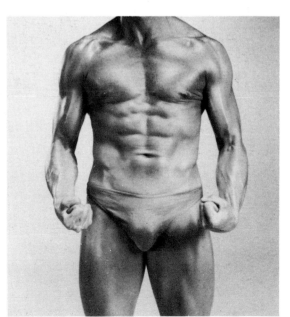

FOREARMS

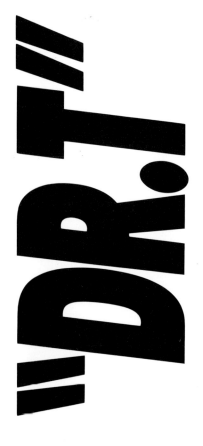

I could see myself skating across the blue line at Maple Leaf Gardens wearing the double-blue uniform with the Maple Leaf on the front and number 7 on the back. This was my goal from early childhood – to play hockey for the Toronto Maple Leafs. A goal which was shattered at age 13 when I fell from a tree into a ravine 20 feet below and landed on my back. Shortly after I started to develop headaches, cold symptoms, stiffness, congestion and irritability. Then I began to have difficulty breathing. The medical doctors diagnosed me as asthmatic, and my career as a hockey player was over because by then I could not keep up with the other players and the exertion would bring on more attacks.

*D*etermined not to quit, ''Never give up'', as my father taught me, I reasoned that since the asthma attacks left me exhausted, and my back and stomach muscles aching, I should exercise those muscles specifically in order to help ward off the attacks. My father bought me my first set of weights when I was 14.

*M*y asthma persisted for ten long years until the day I accompanied my girlfriend to her chiropractic treatment for back injuries she received in a gymnastics accident. It was there that I became interested in chiropractic as a career, and enrolled in the Canadian Memorial Chiropractic College.

*I*n my first year I became a patient at the college clinic for my headaches. Headaches had become a regular part of my life for 10 years, but the frequent pounding in my head made it difficult to read or study. The chiropractor who treated me was delighted that I also had asthma, because he believed that he could also treat that – I was his first asthma patient.

*W*e were both very impressed when after 6 weeks I was able to run 3 miles at a time, where before I could not run across the street without wheezing. That year I played hockey for the first time in 10 years, and began enjoying the athletic activities which had been forbidden for so long. This tremendous recovery cemented my belief in the chiropractic philosophy of subluxation, which means a vertebrae out of alignment with the adjacent vertebrae causes an interference to the nerves which affects the body's ability to function.

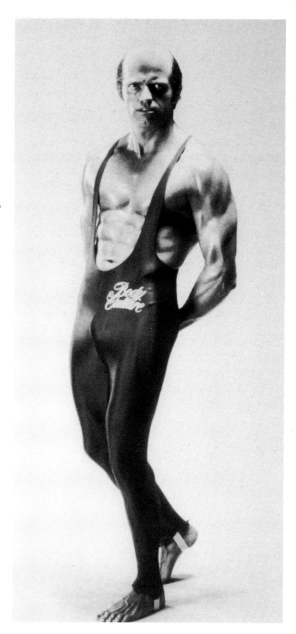

I found out during the course of treatment that the fall I had when I was 13 years old had subluxated several vertebrae in my spine affecting the adrenal gland and lungs which together caused the asthma. The headaches were caused by a subluxation of the cervical area. They were the first to be healed, but the asthma took much longer because of the years of damage to the lungs, but as the attacks became less frequent and severe, I grew stronger and healthier.

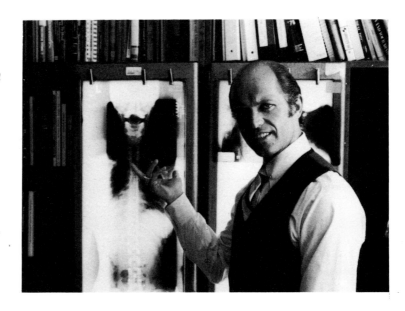

*T*he goal of my initial practice in Toronto was to help asthma and allergy patients who suffered as I had done. I learned quickly that Chiropractic was far more encompassing than just treatment for headaches and asthma. By removing nerve interference countless conditions have been successfully treated. As my practice matured I realized that the results my patients were getting could be improved and maintained if they became interested in exercise and diet to augment their treatment programs.

I initially began creating exercises for specific treatments and would give these out as hand drawn photocopies. As the collection of exercises increased it soon became apparent that they should be displayed in bookform, and this book is a result of those years of work.

*F*itness is a matter of self-motivation. There are many ways to achieve your goals if you "never give in".

*T*o your health,

Roger L. Turner, D.C.

Other recommended reading .

HARD BODIES

HARD IS BEAUTIFUL;
HARD IS SEXY!

*Gladys Portugues and Joyce
Vedral*

*Fitness has come to mean firmness, even
sensual hardness. Soft and loose are out
of vogue, and hard and tight is the
sensuality of the eighties.*

*The best way to ensure a hard body,
shapely muscles, sleek lines and
planned curves is by training with
weights. No other activity can so
effectively resculpt sagging muscles and
develop muscles that keep a woman
looking and feeling young, strong and
healthy.*

*Gladys Portugues and Joyce Vedral
show how to plan your workout routine,
and how to use weights — not to make
you into a professional bodybuilder, but
to give your body its most perfect form.*

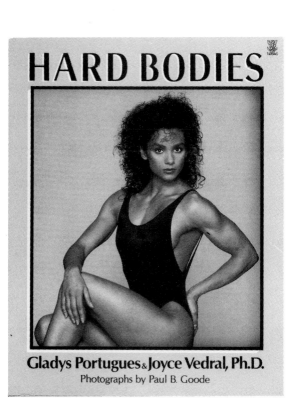

HARD BODIES

Gladys Portugues & Joyce Vedral, Ph.D.
Photographs by Paul B. Goode

SHAPE YOUR BODY
SHAPE YOUR LIFE

THE WEIGHT TRAINING WAY
TO TOTAL FITNESS

Tony **L**ycholat

Weight training — as opposed to weight lifting or body building — is for you, for people of any age, shape or build, to help you to shape your life. Benefits — from strength to aerobic fitness — can be gained from using both free and fixed weight systems in an appropriate and progressive manner. Exercise that produces physical change leads to positive mental changes, too, while increased confidence, reduced anxiety and improved self-esteem frequently partner obvious improvements in body shape and fitness. Here the links between mental and physical health are explained in step with a highly practical guide to training with weights: how to exercise, how to choose equipment and devise a programme to suit your requirements are all explained in this lively and fully illustrated passport to a new you!

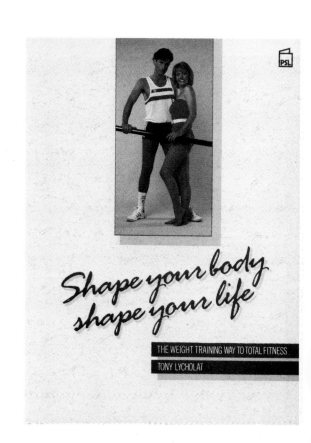

Shape your body
shape your life

THE WEIGHT TRAINING WAY TO TOTAL FITNESS
TONY LYCHOLAT

BODY LOVE

MOVEMENT FOR TOTAL WELL BEING

Peggy Brusseau

"I love you!" When was the last time you said that to your own body?

From the moment you pick up this amazing book you're going to start seeing your body in a revolutionary, new and positive way.

Forget punishing workouts. Stop forcing your body to be something it isn't.

Body Love focuses exclusively on you: your body, your mind and your emotions. These simple movements grow with you and from you, they change and improve as your personality and your potential develop. In this approach, you choose the path of discovery, you design a practice which is unique to you alone.

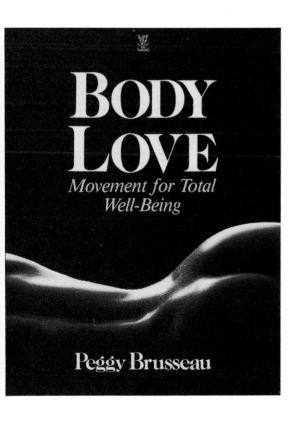

WEIGHT TRAINING FOR MEN

Tony Lycholat

With the current trends in health and fitness many men are now contemplating training with weights to achieve the positive benefits of exercise, yet for the beginner this is a confusing and difficult task. What exactly are the benefits to be gained from weight training? Which method is best? What is Nautilus equipment? Will I become muscle bound?

This book answers all these questions clearly and simply, with numerous explanatory photographs accompanying the text. It illustrates how to design and implement your personal programme, from warming-up through to cooling down so as to achieve health benefits in safety. This book is invaluable to all those embarking upon a weight training programme for the first time, and it also features many useful ideas for the experienced trainer.

Tony Lycholat has an honours degree in Human Movement, specialising in Sportscience from the University of Kent at Canterbury, and is a full member of the British Association of Sport and Medicine and the American College of Sports Medicine. He is also a qualified weight training teacher and athletics coach.

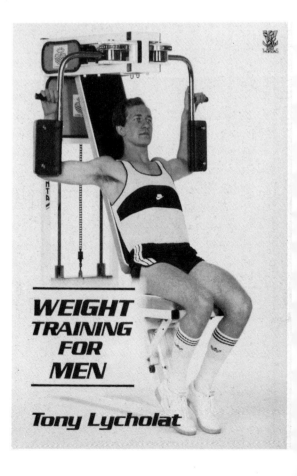

WEIGHT TRAINING FOR MEN

Tony Lycholat

WEIGHT TRAINING FOR WOMEN

Tony Lycholat

*W*ith the current trends in health and fitness many women are now contemplating training with weights to achieve the positive benefits of exercise, yet for the beginner this is a confusing and difficult task. What exactly are the benefits to be gained from weight training? Which method is best? What is Nautilus equipment? Will I become muscle bound? Will I look too masculine?

*T*his book answers all these questions clearly and simply, with numerous explanatory photographs accompanying the text. It illustrates how to design and implement your personal programme, from warming-up through to cooling down so as to achieve health benefits in safety. This book is invaluable to all those embarking upon a weight training programme for the first time, and it also features many useful ideas for the experienced trainer.

*T*ony Lycholat has an honours degree in Human Movement, specialising in Sportscience from the University of Kent at Canterbury, and is a full member of the British Association of Sport and Medicine and the American College of Sports Medicine. He is also a qualified weight training teacher and athletics coach.

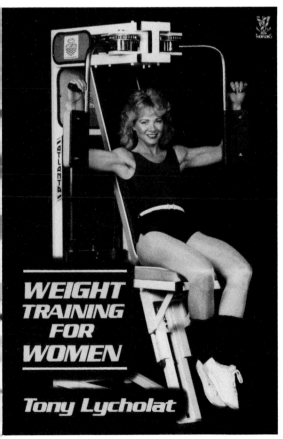

WEIGHT TRAINING FOR WOMEN

Tony Lycholat

FAMILY FITNESS

MUSCLE TONING EXERCISES FOR ALL THE FAMILY

Barbara **R**oberton

The message that fitness is the key to a happy and healthy life is getting through to more and more people — and not just individuals. Whole families are discovering the benefits of regular exercise together. This bright, friendly book, like previous titles in PSL's best-selling fitness series, is designed to encourage and not to cajole and is packed with ideas and exercise routines to get your family fitter. With all members of the family following the programme set out here, there's every incentive to keep going and to benefit from the results.

There's advice about sports and healthy eating, about pastimes beyond the home and about looking and feeling good as individuals and as a family. As the mother of two young children herself, Barbara Roberton, a full-time dance and keep-fit teacher, understands the pressures that families can face and the difficulty of keeping up good intentions. Few families with any interest in health and their own well-being will want to be without this valuable, practical and fully illustrated guide.

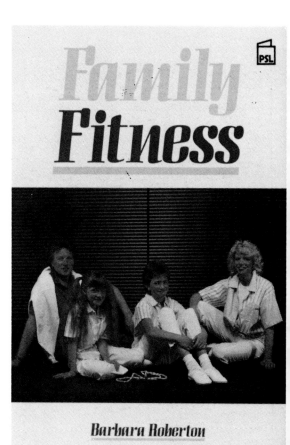

THE JOY OF TOUCH

A GUIDE TO SENSUAL MASSAGE

Russ A. Rueger, Ph.D.

From childhood on, society has allowed us to indulge in the joys of sight, sound, smell and taste; but the most primitive, powerful and tantalizing of all the senses — touch — has always been taboo.

Here is a lavish and fully illustrated guidebook to that neglected sense. This uninhibited celebration of the human body shows us how to use our hands, lips, tongue, hair and nose to evoke everything in our partners from laughter to goosepimple eroticism.

Discover the full spectrum of sensuous massage techniques, the magic of healing through touching, touch for stimulation and well-being and even touch enhancers.

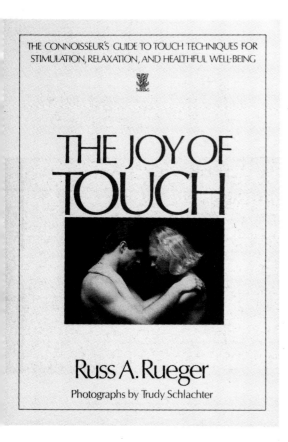

PATRICK STEPHENS LIMITED

Patrick Stephens have published authoritative, quality books for enthusiasts for more than twenty years. During that time they have established a reputation as one of the world's leading publishers of books on aviation, maritime, military, model making, motor cycling, motoring, motor racing, railway and railway modelling subjects as well as health and fitness.

    In 1984, PSL became part of the Thorsons Publishing Group, since when significant further expansion of the Company's publishing programme has continued to take place.

    If you would like a free catalogue describing the present range of PSL titles, please write to:

Patrick Stephens Limited
Wellingborough
Northamptonshire, NN8 2QD